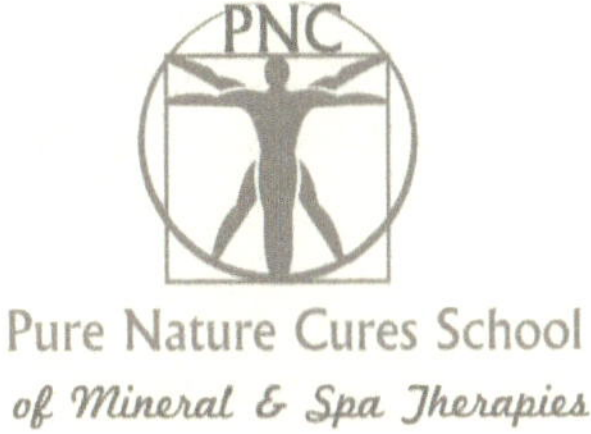

Far Infrared Mineral Weight Loss Wrap Course for Clinic & Home Use

Learn how to use clays, salts and far infrared for sustainable weight loss and better health

Galina St George

Table of Contents

Disclaimer

The author of this material sincerely believes that a natural approach to health and maintaining a natural balance within the human body are very important in experiencing energy, vitality, and vibrant health throughout life.

The author recognizes that opinions within scientific and medical fields differ greatly. The purpose of this book is to share educational information and scientific research gathered by the author, scientists, and informed advocates of health and well-being using natural methods and resources.

None of the information contained in this book is intended to diagnose, prevent, treat, or cure any disease, nor is it intended to prescribe any of the techniques, materials or concepts presented as a form of treatment for any illness or medical condition. Before beginning any practice pertaining to procedures described in the book, it is highly recommended that you first obtain the consent and advice of a licensed health care professional.

The information given in this book should be used for educational purposes only, and not as advice or prescription for specific medical conditions. Responsibility for any action taken as a result of reading this book will lie solely with you. The author assumes no responsibility for the choices you make after your review of the information contained herein and your consultation with a licensed healthcare professional.

Also, if you are on medication, do not start taking or using minerals without your doctor's permission, since being powerful sorbents, clays can interfere with medicines.

Introduction

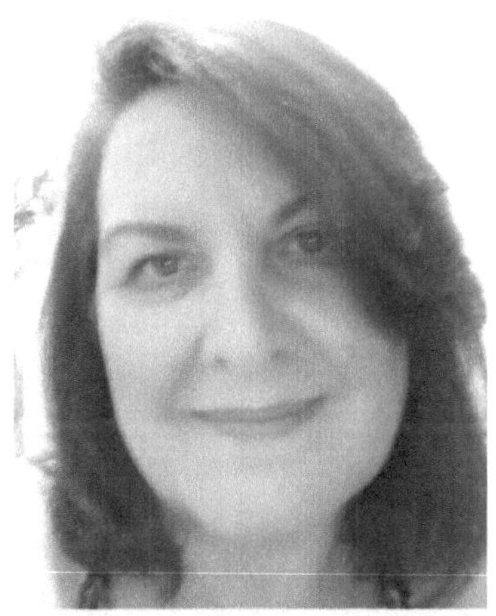

Weight loss is possibly one of the most painful and widely discussed subjects in all parts of the world. Why have we found ourselves in the situation we are in? The problem is not just present in the Western world.

The statistics show that a vast number of people in the developing world are suffering from various degrees of obesity which has led to a concern being repeatedly expressed by the World Health Organisation at least for two decades.

However, I guess it's a rhetorical question since there are many reasons for it – social, psychological, environmental and so on. It is not the purpose of this course to analyse them since to cover such reasons would require writing a separate book.

The focus of this course is on sustainable weight loss through mineral supplementation, detox, lymphatic drainage, improved circulation and metabolism due to the healing factors created by far-infrared and minerals.

The treatment was created by myself based on years of research into healing powers of minerals which I have been using for many years. I love clay. It's simple and yet so potent. I love other minerals as well and have written a lot about their healing properties which are widely used by spas worldwide.

So about 12 years ago I created a range of mineral-based treatments which I have been practising on my clients.

Having devised the treatment I decided to create a course to train others in what I have learned over the years about this wonderful mineral and also to help better understand how clays worked and how they can be used to help us live healthier lives.

It is important to mention that the printed or Kindle versions of the course do not include certification. To get certified, you will need to take the online version with the quizzes, case studies, assignments and the final assessment. This book aims to introduce the idea of healing with clays and far-infrared and also to complement the online course.

Galina St George

Module 1 - Course Overview: Resources, Certification, Materials and Equipment, Disclaimer and Therapist Qualification Requirements.

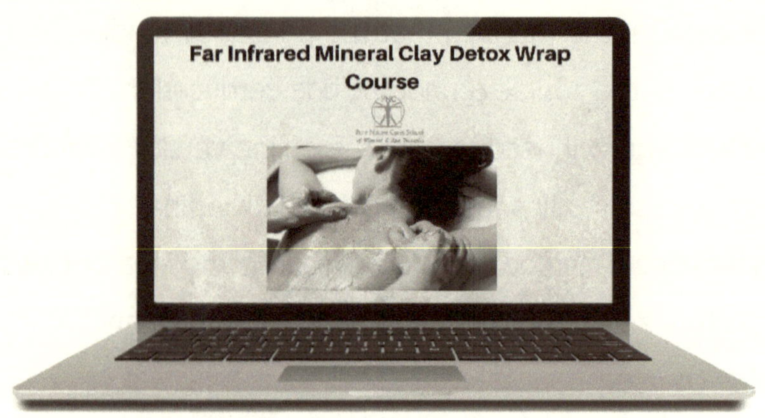

Unit 1 – Course Overview: Resources, Certification and Other Details

Course Overview

Far Infrared Clay Detox Course is one of a range of courses developed by Pure Nature Cures School of Mineral & Spa Therapies. The course explores multiple health benefits of magnesium and various transdermal applications of magnesium salts.

Who Is This Course Suitable For?

1. Therapists with a valid Level 3 Anatomy & Physiology + Massage qualifications – to obtain professional insurance and be able to practice professionally.

2. Members of the public who would like to learn the course for their benefit.

Resources

1. Course units

2. Recommended literature & websites.

Certification

The course has been approved by the International Institute of Holistic Therapists. Certification is issued by the Pure Nature Cures School of Mineral & Spa Therapies.

To get certified, you will need to go through our online course and complete the test questions after corresponding units.

Everyone who has completed the course units and quizzes will be issued with a certificate of completion.

If you decide to qualify as a therapist, you will need to complete an add-on unit for therapists, case studies, the practical module and assignments. This will qualify you for the practitioner certificate which you can use to apply for professional insurance.

You will need to make enquiries with your local insurance providers to obtain professional insurance.

Materials & Equipment Needed for the Treatment

1. Clay – calcium bentonite, green montmorillonite, green illite, white kaolin
2. Water
3. Far Infrared Blanket
4. Plastic sheet
5. Large bowl
6. Spatula
7. Other components will be described later in the course.

Unit 2 – Disclaimer

Medical Disclaimer

Neither I personally nor my business makes any representations or guarantees in terms of medical information and research materials described in this Course, express or implied. All information in this Course is presented solely for educational purposes, and not to diagnose or treat any person for any medical symptom, illness or condition.

None of the information, treatments and techniques presented in this Course, in written or oral communication, within our Practical modules, webinars and consultations aims to replace or teach to replace medical diagnosis or treatment. Students are always encouraged to seek medical diagnosis and treatment for any medical problems.

While we aim to present what we believe to be complete, accurate and true information, considering a diversity of views in the medical research field, we cannot guarantee that the information in this Course is always complete, accurate and true. This does exempt us from any liabilities and responsibilities which may not be excluded by applicable legislation.

It is a responsibility of the Reader/ Student/ Therapist to assess their own or their client's health and to make an appropriate decision regarding the suitability of advice or treatment in each particular case. Written consent of the 3rd party must always be obtained before any advice or treatment is provided.

We list some contra-indications to the treatments described in our course materials. However, the list is not exhaustive. The Reader/ Student/ Therapist must always make their assessment of any conditions the 3rd party presents them with and decide as to whether a treatment is appropriate for themselves or their client.

We will not be held responsible for 3rd party decisions, consultations, treatments or results of these which happen outside the premises and assigned time schedule of the Practical Module Course.

Professional Advice Disclaimer

Neither the information contained within this Course nor communication between the Course Provider/ Book Author/ Business on one hand and Reader/ Student/ Therapist on the other hand, in any form or on any subject – such as medicine, pharmacology, psychology, finances, commerce, marketing, taxes, accounting, must be regarded nor used as a substitution for professional advice.

Earnings Disclaimer

Neither the information on this Website nor digital or other forms of communication between the Reader/ Student/ Therapist aim to offer any guarantees in terms of potential earnings.

You accept that financial and another type of success depend on a variety of factors, such as knowledge, skills, abilities, dedication, experience, strategies, marketing efforts, networking, the spending power of your potential clients, etc.

As a professional therapist, you are the only person responsible for your earnings and financial success. While we outline revenue potential as a result of the skills you have learned with us, we cannot give any promises or guarantees in this respect, and no statements on this website aim to mislead you in this respect.

Persons under 16

Persons under 16 years of age require their parent's permission to use materials, treatments and techniques, as well as to receive a consultation or a treatment described in this Course. It is the responsibility of a Reader/ Student/ Therapist to ensure that such permission has been obtained before a consultation or a treatment has been provided to a person who is under 16 years of age.

Personal & Professional Responsibility

You agree that you are solely responsible for your own professional (public, product and any other relevant type) liability as a result of your actions. You are the only person responsible for your compliance with the law and regulations in any area of your business.

You agree that by using this Course information and Services, you take full responsibility for your own decisions, actions and results of your actions towards yourself or 3rd parties. You agree to comply with laws and legislation of the country you live in. You are solely responsible for your Professional Indemnlty Insurance, National Insurance and taxes.

We highly recommend that you make enquiries about membership of professional organisations and professional liability insurance before you start treating clients. You should always work in the interests of your clients (paying or non-paying) and within the framework of legal and ethical considerations.

All the courses and treatments presented by Pure Nature Cures School of Mineral & Spa Therapies are being marketed as complementary health and beauty courses and treatments, and are not meant to promote or endorse any medical information, or provide diagnosis and/or medical treatment.

Contraindications to Treatments

If you have any medical condition, please address it with a medical professional. The treatments have certain contra-indications, so are not suitable for everyone. See the list of common contra-indications and cautions here:

https://courses.purenaturecures.com/contraindications-cautions.

There may be other conditions not listed here which may make a person unsuitable for treatment. If you are unsure, please refer your client to a medical professional. Never conduct treatment without prior consultation to establish a client's suitability for the procedure.

Pure Nature Cures School of Mineral & Spa Therapies offers no diagnosis or treatment of problems of a medical nature, and no guarantees in terms of health benefits described within the Course.

While there are multiple possible benefits to the treatments, they should be seen as part of the integrative approach to health issues rather than a sole option. Any positive results will depend on a combination of factors taken by you or your client, and we cannot and do not offer any guarantees in terms of benefits mentioned within our offers or the course syllabus.

Please let us know if you have any questions, and we will be happy to reply. You can contact us by email: **support@purenaturecures.com**.

For more detailed information about the terms and conditions of using our website and training please see https://courses.purenaturecures.com/terms/

Unit 3 - Therapist Qualification Requirements

The courses run by the Pure Nature Cures School of Mineral & Spa Therapies are aimed both at therapists and members of the public.

- Members of the public take our courses to learn about the health benefits of salts, clays and minerals and do treatments on themselves, based on their assessment of their health. In the case of existing health issues, members of the public should always seek medical advice before having a treatment. Even though the majority of people will benefit from the treatments, some people may find them unsuitable.

- Our courses can also be taken by qualified therapists who would like to add new skills to their portfolio. To be considered qualified, a therapist needs to have a Level 3 Anatomy & Physiology and Body Massage Diploma.

- While all the students will be issued with the Certificate of Completion, only qualified therapists will receive a Practitioner Certificate which will allow them to apply for Practitioner insurance and treat members of the public.

- We cannot guarantee that the qualification we offer will be accepted by insurers in the country of your residence, due to variations regarding requirements for complementary therapies. Please make enquiries with your local insurance providers.

- To qualify as a therapist, you will need to sign up for the add-on short course for therapists which covers subjects such as hygiene, professional issues, as well as case studies.

- The optional practical one-day module is offered to therapists in the UK & Northern Ireland, as well as to those who can travel to the UK for the course.

Module 2 - Excess Weight and Obesity. BMI - Body Mass Index. Causes and Health Risks of Obesity.

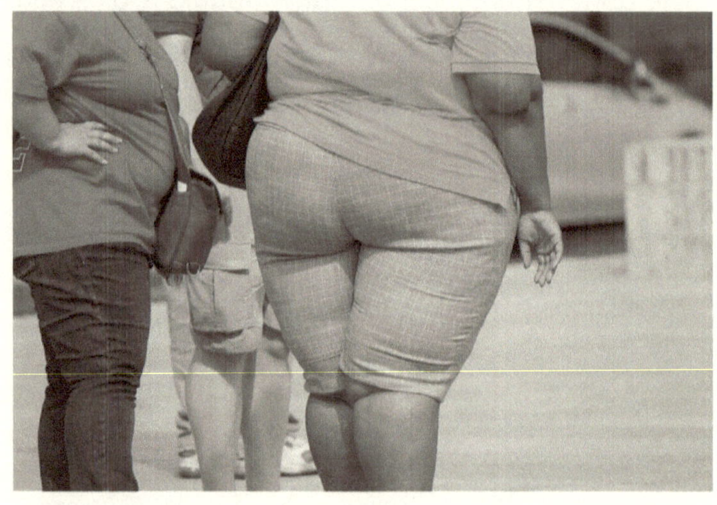

Unit 1 - Excess Weight and Obesity - Facts and Figures

Key Statistics

- According to the World Health Organisation (WHO), the number of obese people has tripled worldwide since 1975.
- Obesity and excess weight kill more people worldwide than hunger and being underweight.
- 39% of adults were overweight and 13% obese in 2016.
- 340 million children and adolescents under the age of 5-19 were obese in 2016.
- 41 million children under the age of 5 were overweight in the same year.

What is obesity?

"Obesity is the heavy accumulation of fat in your body to such a degree that it significantly increases your risk of diseases that can damage your health and knock years off your life, such as heart disease and diabetes. The fat may be equally distributed around the body or concentrated around the abdomen or midriff (apple-shaped) or the hips and thighs (pear-shaped)."

http://www.netdoctor.co.uk/health_advice/facts/obesity.ht
m

Overweight vs obese

The difference between the two is in the BMI (we will talk
about it in the follow-up units).
If the BMI is 25 or over, a person is classified as
overweight.
If the BMI is 30 or over, a person is classified as obese.

More statistics

- Excess weight and obesity are the 5th leading risk
  for global deaths.
- According to the WHO, at least 2.8 million adults die
  each year as a result of being overweight or obese.
- 44% of diabetes, 23% of the ischaemic heart
  disease and between 7% and 41% of certain

cancers are connected with excess weight and obesity.

- 65% of the world's population live in countries where excess weight and obesity kill more people than underweight (this includes all high-income and most middle-income countries.
- By 2050 the prevalence of obesity is predicted to affect 60% of adult men, 50% of adult women.

Further Reading

1. Obesity Facts & Figures. http://easo.org/obesity-facts-figures
2. Obesity in Adults.
http://www.patient.co.uk/doctor/obesity-in-adults
4. The Link between Obesity, Cancer & Toxicity.
http://www.naturalnews.com/022804_cancer_obesity_fat.html

Unit 2 - Body Mass Index (BMI)

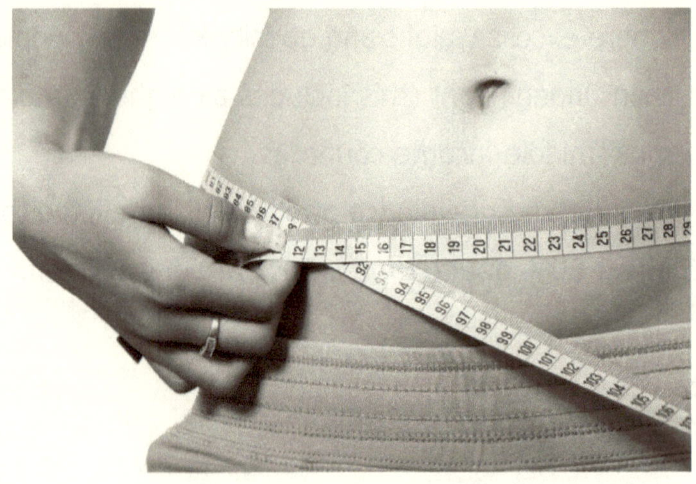

BMI, which stands for the Body Mass Index, is the weight in kilograms divided by the square of the height in meters (kg/m2). It is a commonly used index to classify underweight, normal and excessive weight and obesity in adults.

The World Health Organisation defines being overweight as a BMI equal to or more than 25 and being obese when a

BMI goes over 30.

The full classification of BMI:

- <18.5 - underweight
- 18.5 - 24.9 - normal weight
- >25 - overweight
- 25 - 29.5 - pre-obese
- >30 - obese
- 30 - 34.9 - moderately obese (class I)
- 35 - 39.9 - severely obese (class II)
- >40 - very severely obese (class III)
- >45 - morbidly obese (class IV)
- >50 - super obese (class V)
- >55 - hyper-obese(Class VI).

It is important to remember that the BMI figures apply to adults - not to children or adolescents. To learn more about these groups and which are classified as overweight and obese, see the WHO website.

The other thing that should be noted is that the BMI is only a rough indicator of obesity and excess weight. People who are into sport and fitness may have a high BMI but will not be considered obese or even overweight due to the fact that muscles are denser and heavier than fat. So, a weight lifter or a bodybuilder with a large muscle bulk cannot be put into the same group as a person of the same BMI who does little or no exercise.

Women and men would be classified differently because of the average differences in the muscle bulk and bone density.

There are also regional variations too. For example, in Hong Kong, a person of 25-30 BMI would be considered overweight/moderately obese and a BMI of 30 would qualify a person as morbidly obese. In Japan, there are simply 4 levels of obesity, with the 4th level being the highest.

While the BMI remains relevant as a rough guide to what is seen as normal, it is important not to follow it to the letter for the reasons already mentioned here.

In 1998, the US National Institutes of Health and Centres for Disease Control and Prevention brought US definitions in line with the WHO guidelines - from 27.8 to 25, and overnight 29 million Americans were reclassified from healthy to obese. So, these numbers should be seen as a guideline only. Other factors like a person's fitness level, muscle to fat ratio and general health should certainly be taken into account.

Unit 3 – What Causes Obesity?

The basic cause of obesity is energy imbalance where consumed calories exceed the calories spent. This leads to the storage of unspent energy in the body tissues - the main body parts like the trunk, arms, legs, the head as well as in the internal organs such as the liver, heart and kidneys.

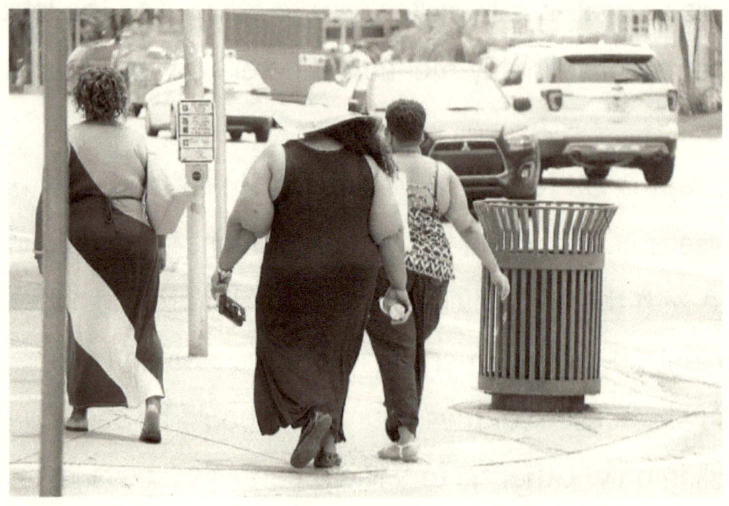

Following are the most common causes of obesity:

- Eating more than your body spends on life processes and activities
- Eating food poor in nutrients
- Eating food which is high in refined carbohydrates, fats and artificial food additives
- Eating food which is low in fibre

- Eating foods which are loaded with artificial additives - they are common disruptors of hormonal balance in the body
- Being exposed to environmental toxins (these get into the body from water, food and air, and include man-produced toxins, heavy metals, by-products of the pharmaceutical industry, plastics, pesticides, fertilisers, hormones)
- Low daily physical activity
- Sedentary lifestyle
- Chronic stress
- Insufficient sleep on a regular basis
- Snacking frequently on high-calorie food
- Prescription medications - corticosteroids, antidepressants, contraceptives - these are all disruptive for the hormone system.
- Many other medications
- Toxins used in preservatives and other food additives
- Alcohol abuse.

These are the main causes of excess weight and obesity

but not all. Some of these causes have underlying factors. For example, alcohol and substance abuse, overeating and sedentary lifestyle may be connected to psychological motives such as depression, low self-esteem stemming from childhood trauma or stressful life events.

A job of a weight loss practitioner is to find out as much as he or she can during a consultation and refer the client to an appropriate therapist - be it a mental health practitioner such as a counsellor/ psychologist or a general health practitioner who can refer the client further.

A weight loss practitioner should never try to deal with the issues they are not qualified to address.

Unit 4 - Health Risks of Obesity

Obesity can cause or be associated with:

- Breathlessness

- Snoring
- Fatigue
- Type 2 diabetes
- Colon cancer
- Hypertension
- Raised cholesterol levels
- Stroke
- Coronary heart disease
- Increased risk of a heart attack
- Increases the risk of other types of cancer
- Gallstones
- Kidney disease
- Osteoarthritis
- Back and joint pain
- Increased risk of infertility
- Pregnancy complications (pre-eclampsia, eclampsia, gestational diabetes)
- Increased risk of impotence
- Varicose veins
- Reduced life expectancy
- Psychological issues such as low confidence and

depression

- Cancer.

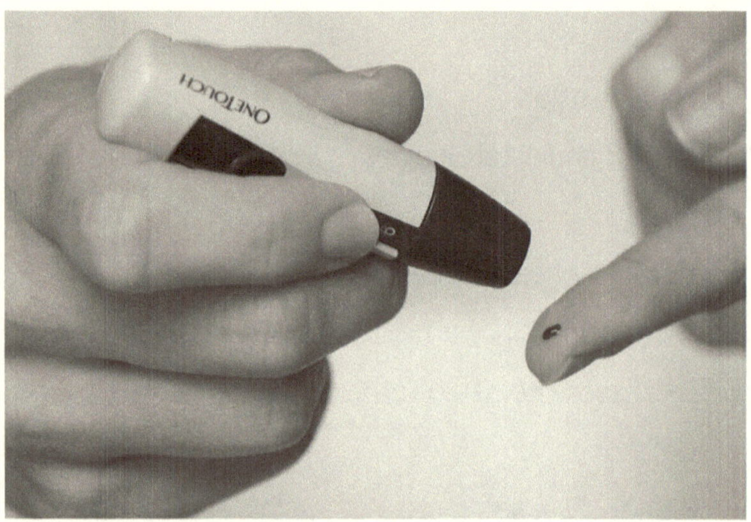

Not everyone who is overweight develops these problems. The risks rise where there is a family history of any of the above conditions. Also, the distribution of weight around the body plays an important part in this. For example, if the fat is mostly found around the waistline the possibility of developing associated health conditions increases dramatically.

Losing excess weight lowers the chances of developing health problems. However, losing weight too fast can cause complications in certain cases. For example, it can aggravate the cases of gout and gallstones. Gradual weight loss of 1-2 pounds a week is a much healthier way to achieve the desired result and, above all, maintain it.

Further reading

What Are the Health Risks of Obesity?
http://www.bbc.co.uk/science/0/21702372

Module 3 - The Role of Environmental Toxins in Developing Obesity. Detoxification Methods.

Unit 1 - The Role of Environmental Toxins in Developing Obesity and Diabetes.

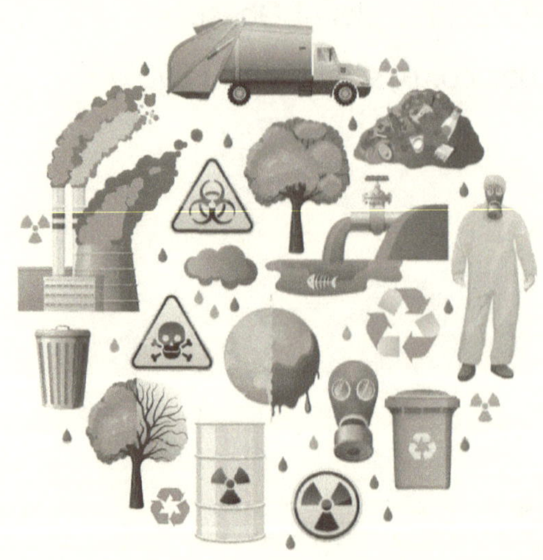

The fast growth in the rate of obesity and type II diabetes

in the past few decades has prompted scientists to look into possible causes which extend beyond diet and exercise. Various scientific research experiments have been conducted to establish the link, with very interesting results.

"Exposure to environmental toxins in the absence of increased caloric intake induces weight gain and insulin resistance. Stated simply, toxins are an invisible, unappreciated cause of obesity and diabetes...

The most recent example of how toxins induce obesity is the dramatic increase in obesity in babies. In 2006, scientists at the Harvard School of Public Health found that rates of obesity in infants less than 6 months old have risen 73% since 1980. This epidemic of obesity in 6-month-olds is not related to diet or lack of exercise. It appears it may be a load of environmental toxins in their little bodies...

Mounting evidence points to a unique and unappreciated trigger for obesity - exposure to small traces of environmental chemicals in the environment. The average new-born has 287 chemicals in the umbilical cord blood, 217 of which are neurotoxic. The chemicals these infants are exposed to include pesticides, phthalates, bisphenol A, flame retardants, and heavy metals such as mercury, lead, and arsenic 11. These chemicals have a broad range of negative effects on human biology. They are neurotoxic, carcinogenic, and now it seems, obesogenic."

http://drhyman.com/downloads/Diabetes-and-Toxins.pdf

Here is some more data which can be used as proof that exposure to environmental toxins is closely linked to obesity and type II diabetes:

"Data from the government's National Health and Nutrition Examination Survey 1999-2002 found a very striking correlation between blood levels of six common persistent organic pollutants (petrochemical toxins) and diabetes. Those who had the highest serum levels of pollutants had a dramatically higher risk for diabetes."

http://drhyman.com/downloads/Diabetes-and-Toxins.pdf

"A 2008 study in JAMA found that bisphenol A, a petrochemical that lines water bottles and canned food containers, increases the risk of diabetes, heart disease, and abnormal liver function." Source

"Canadian Aboriginals and Great Lakes sports fishermen both have higher rates of diabetes from eating contaminated seafood. The ubiquitous exposure to persistent organic pollutants (POPs) such as diphenyl dichloroethene (DDE), polychlorinated biphenyls (PCBs), and polybrominated diphenyl ethers (PBDEs) have been linked to obesity and diabetes."
http://drhyman.com/downloads/Diabetes-and-Toxins.pdf

"The burgeoning obesity epidemic has placed enormous strains on individual and societal health mandating a careful search for pathogenic factors, including the contributions made by endocrine disrupting chemicals (EDCs). In addition to evidence that some exogenous chemicals have the capacity to modulate classical hormonal signalling axes, there is mounting evidence that several EDCs can also disrupt metabolic pathways and alter energy homeostasis. Adipose tissue appears to be a particularly important target of these metabolic disruptions.

A diverse array of compounds has been shown to alter adipocyte differentiation, and several EDCs have been shown to modulate adipocyte physiology, including adipocytic insulin action and adipokine secretion. This rapidly emerging evidence demonstrating that environmental contaminants alter adipocyte function emphasizes the potential role that disruption of adipose physiology by EDCs may play in the global epidemic of metabolic disease."
http://www.sciencedirect.com/science/article/pii/S0925443913001907

"These toxins are not only obesogens but also carcinogens and autogens, which trigger autoimmune and inflammatory disorders and cardiovascular mortality. They are also neurotoxic and have been linked to increased rates of

depression, autism spectrum disorders, attention deficit disorder, and dementia."
http://link.springer.com/article/10.1007%2Fs13679-014-0094-y

"The "chemical obesogen" hypothesis conjectures that synthetic, environmental contaminants are contributing to the global epidemic of obesity. In fact, intentional food additives (e.g., artificial sweeteners and colours, emulsifiers) and unintentional compounds (e.g., bisphenol A, pesticides) are largely unstudied in regard to their effects on overall metabolic homeostasis. With that said, many of these contaminants have been found to dysregulate endocrine function, insulin signalling, and/or adipocyte function."
http://link.springer.com/article/10.1007%2Fs13679-014-0094-y

See more scientific data here -
http://online.liebertpub.com/doi/abs/10.1089/10755530231 7371479

We could continue citing the results of various scientific experiments and research, but this may be sufficient to make a conclusion that toxins we get from food and the environment indeed contribute towards disruption of metabolic activity.

This doesn't mean that we should all just accept that the environment is the reason for our being overweight/ obese. It just sheds some light on this complex issue. To deal with obesity effectively, we need to study its possible causes. Lack of exercise, over-eating, and eating junk food still take the first place as the main causes of obesity. However, it is important to look at a range of factors to establish them.

Further Reading

1. Diabetes and Toxins, Dr Hyman.
http://drhyman.com/downloads/Diabetes-and-Toxins.pdf

2. Adipocytes under assault: Environmental disruption of adipose physiology.

http://www.sciencedirect.com/science/article/pii/S0925443
913001907

3. Increased methylmercury toxicity related to obesity in diabetic KK-Ay mice.

http://www.ncbi.nlm.nih.gov/pubmed/24243536

Unit 2 - Traditional Detoxification Methods

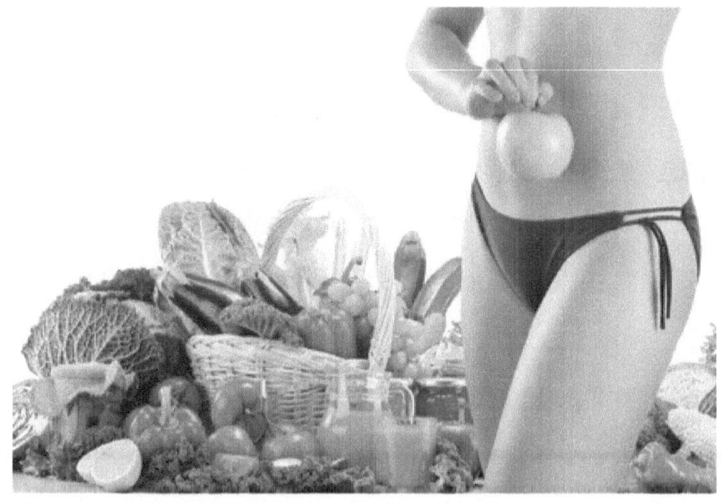

Following are the most common detoxification methods:

Diet and nutrition. Introduce phytonutrients into your diet. This includes Brussels sprouts, Bok Choi, wasabi, kale, coriander, turnips, curcumin, radishes, watercress, cabbage, cauliflower, garlic, onions. Most of these contain sulphur which binds many toxins in the body. Also, eat eggs and other protein-based foods. Drink green tea (increases glutathione-s-transferases, contains antioxidants).

Supplementation. "The most critical endogenous molecule for detoxification is glutathione. Optimal methylation is required to generate glutathione through the methylation/transsulfuration cycle, making B6, folic acid, and B12 essential. Zinc and selenium also facilitate detoxification as cofactors in the enzymes metallothionein and glutathione peroxidase. N-acetyl-cysteine increases glutathione and historically has been used to treat depleted glutathione and liver failure from acetaminophen overdose. Milk thistle has long been used in liver disease and increases glutathione. Buffered ascorbic acid (vitamin C) is also critical in detoxification and has been associated with a reduction in lead levels."

href="http://drhyman.com/downloads/Diabetes-and-Toxins.pdf

Sun Chlorella, spirulina - these are rich in a number of phytonutrients which have been researched for their detoxifying properties and shown to bind heavy metals and other environmental toxins.

Chelation therapy - a medical procedure which involves the binding of heavy metals such as arsenic, mercury, lead, etc, using various chemical agents. This is performed over a course of time in a hospital environment in cases of serious toxicity.

Sauna therapy. "The Environmental Protection Agency has shown that sauna therapy increases the excretion of heavy metals (lead; mercury; cadmium; and fat-soluble chemicals such as PCBs, PBBs, and HCBs)."

http://drhyman.com/downloads/Diabetes-and-Toxins.pdf

Physical exercise. Physical activity promotes circulation and sweating which helps to move toxins out of the body better than many other methods. In order to ensure a regular and timely removal of toxins, we should ensure that we exercise regularly. It is important to remember that although strenuous exercise has a great impact on toxin removal it is even more important to be consistently active. Taking a daily 30-minute walk is a great way to exercise even if you can't or won't go to a gym.

Massage is an excellent way to help move toxins out of the body due to its stimulating, blood and lymph moving effects. While any form of body massage is good for this, there is a specific type which serves this purpose best - Manual Lymph Drainage. A therapist doing it will be working very gently and slowly to help move the lymph in the right direction.

Reflexology is another therapy which helps to reduce toxicity. By gently stimulating the foot or hand reflexes (some reflexologists work on other body parts like the ears), a therapist will be promoting blood circulation and lymph flow which is a powerful way of getting toxins out of the body.

These are just some most common and well-known detoxification methods and there are many others.

Module 4 - Link Between Stress and Obesity

Unit 1 - Types of Stress, Common Symptoms and Consequences

We are used to common thinking that when we get stressed, we lose appetite, and therefore weight. Well, yes and no. The relationship between stress and obesity is a lot more complex than this. To understand it, we need to look at the nature of 3 different types of stress, and how they affect the body.

In simple terms, stress is the body-mind response to real or perceived events and situations in its surroundings. It can be caused both by what is perceived as "good" or "bad". The "good" factors include what we find exciting, stimulating, highly pleasurable.

For example, a jump from the plane with a parachute - it is a stressful activity, but in most cases exciting at the same time. The "bad" stressors are the ones which cause distress to the mind and body - for example, an attack - real or imagined, physical or psychological.

Acute Stress

This is a short-lived type of stress. The body responds to it with a "fight or flight" strategy. This kind of response causes fast changes in the body, to ensure its survival. A release of adrenaline and other related hormones mobilises the body resources within a short period of time.

The limb muscles contract, the heart starts pumping the blood a lot faster, blood flow to the limbs and major organs increases, to make sure that the body can either fight or flee. This is a biological response which in dangerous situations saves lives.

However, in many cases danger is perceived, rather than present, and a lot of people get acutely stressed over things which are non-life-threatening (e.g. road rage). Acute stress is accountable for most cases of cardiac arrest (heart attack) and can be very dangerous if there are long-term chronic problems present in the body.

The other type of acute stress involves pleasant activities and events - a birth of a child, moving home, doing something for fun and excitement (e.g. a ski jump). This stress is short-lived, but can still disrupt the body processes.

Common symptoms and consequences:

- A sudden rise in blood pressure
- Muscle tension, cramps
- Disruption of digestive processes
- Increased risk of cardiac arrest
- Increased risk of stroke
- Flaring up of chronic conditions
- Long-term physical and psychological problems.

Repeated acute stress

This kind of stress involves repetition of stressful situations and events on a recurring basis. It also describes the mind's perception of the environment as threatening and hostile, with the corresponding reaction.

Like with acute stress, it can be real (e.g. a soldier or a civilian in a war zone), or perceived (a teenager seeing the world as a deeply hostile environment, with no way out).

This is a more dangerous kind of stress since the body and mind balance get repeatedly disrupted, with hormones wreaking havoc with the body systems.

Common symptoms and consequences:

- Anxiety
- Wearing down of all body systems
- Build-up of toxins in the body
- Stroke
- Cardiac problems
- Cardiac arrest
- Stroke.

Chronic Stress

This is the most dangerous type of stress since it is destroying the body and mind consistently over a period of time.

The most possible causes are the financial hardship, relationship problems, a feeling of being stuck in the rut due to entrenched beliefs and inflexible mindset, long-term illness - of yourself or a family member, lack of help, loneliness, bullying, uninspiring environment - at home or at work.

The damage which long-term stress causes to the body is often devastating. People who are continually exposed to chronic stress are much more likely to suffer from poor health, which leads to a low lifespan.

Common symptoms and consequences

- High cholesterol level in the blood, leading to clogged up and rigid arteries (atherosclerosis and arteriosclerosis)
- Over-eating, leading to obesity
- Obesity caused by the accumulation of toxins in the body

- Type 2 diabetes due to insulin resistance from the cells
- Inflammation of the joints (arthritis, rheumatism)
- Blood pressure abnormalities
- Chronic anxiety
- Depression
- Passive aggression
- Sudden seemingly unexplained episodes of a panic attack and acute anxiety
- Chronic Fatigue Syndrome
- Fibromyalgia
- Kidney disease
- Psoriasis, dermatitis, eczema
- Acne and other skin problems
- Allergies
- Stroke
- Poor immunity
- Disturbed sleep
- Headaches, migraine
- Depression
- Alcoholism

- Drug abuse
- Other addictions
- Cancer.

Further Reading

1. Chronic stress and obesity: A new view of "comfort food". http://www.pnas.org/content/100/20/11696.short
2. Chronic stress, glucocorticoids, insulin and obesity, Mary Dallman.
http://www.endocrine-abstracts.org/ea/0019/ea0019s10.htm
3. Magnesium Deficiency Is Associated with Insulin Resistance in Obese Children, Milagros di Huerta, MD et al.
http://care.diabetesjournals.org/content/28/5/1175.short

Unit 2 - The Link between Stress and Obesity

The relationship between stress and obesity has been established not only by observing human but animal behaviour as well.

It is a well-known fact that while for most of us acute stress doesn't invoke comfort eating, chronic stress does. Why is it happening, and what are the long-term consequences of chronic stress?

Here are conclusions of **2 scientific studies** which explain what happens in the body as a result of chronic stress, and how it leads to obesity:

1. "The effects of adrenal corticosteroids on subsequent adrenocorticotropin secretion are complex. Acutely (within hours), glucocorticoids (GCs) directly inhibit further activity in the hypothalamo–pituitary–adrenal axis, but the chronic actions (across days) of these steroids on the brain are directly excitatory. **Chronically high concentrations of GCs act in three ways** that are functionally congruent.

(i) GCs increase the expression of corticotropin-releasing factor (CRF) mRNA in the central nucleus of the amygdala, a critical node in the emotional brain. CRF enables recruitment of a chronic stress-response network.

(ii) GCs increase the salience of pleasurable or compulsive activities (ingesting sucrose, fat, and drugs, or wheel-running). This motivates ingestion of "comfort food."

(iii) GCs act systemically to increase abdominal fat depots. This allows an increased signal of abdominal energy stores to inhibit catecholamines in the brainstem and CRF expression in hypothalamic neurons regulating adrenocorticotropin.
...In stressed or depressed humans chronic stress induces either increased comfort food intake and body weight gain or decreased intake and body weight loss...

Depressed people who overeat have decreased cerebrospinal CRF, catecholamine concentrations, and hypothalamo–pituitary–adrenal activity. We propose that people eat comfort food in an attempt to reduce the activity in the chronic stress-response network with its attendant anxiety..."

http://www.pnas.org/content/100/20/11696.short

2. "Although stressors generally reduce the intake of boring but healthy foods (chow for rats), both acute and repeated restraint stress increase the intake of highly palatable calories (32% sucrose, lard), when they are available. This behavioural effect is mediated by elevated glucocorticoids and depends on the accompanying increase in circulating insulin concentrations.

In the periphery, whereas glucocorticoids mobilize stored calories and greatly increase the rate of gluconeogenesis, **insulin counteracts the effects of glucocorticoids, abetting caloric storage**. Together, increasing concentrations of both hormones increase adipose storage, at the expense of peripheral protein stores when there is not an overall gain in body weight. " http://www.endocrine-abstracts.org/ea/0019/ea0019s10.htm

3. "In population studies, **adrenal hormones show strong statistical associations to centralization of body fat as well as to obesity**. There is considerable evidence from clinical to cellular and molecular studies that **elevated cortisol**, particularly when combined with secondary inhibition of sex steroids and growth hormone secretions, **is causing accumulation of fat in visceral adipose tissues as well as metabolic abnormalities** (The Metabolic Syndrome). Hypertension is probably due to parallel activation of the central sympathetic nervous system...

Glucocorticoid exposure is also followed by increased food intake and 'leptin resistant' obesity, perhaps disrupting the balance between leptin and neuropeptide Y to the advantage of the latter. The consequence might be **'stress-eating'**, which, however, is a poorly defined entity.

Factors activating the stress centres in humans include psychosocial and socio-economic handicaps, depressive and anxiety traits, alcohol and smoking, with some differences in profile between personalities and genders. Polymorphisms have been defined in several genes associated with the cascade of events along the stress axes."

https://onlinelibrary.wiley.com/doi/abs/10.1046/j.1467-789x.2001.00027.x

4. "Stress is experienced by animals and humans daily and many individuals experience cycles of stress and recovery throughout the day. If we consume larger and less frequent meals, the conditions are favourable for weight gain, especially in the abdomen. We know that belly fat, as well as stress, contributes to the development of **cardiovascular disease, immune dysfunction and other metabolic disorders.**"

http://www.the-aps.org/mm/hp/Audiences/Public-Press/For -the-Press/releases/10/27.html

Unit 3 - Ways of Dealing with Stress

To deal with stress effectively, it is important to identify what's causing it and follow through with an effective and realistic stress management strategy.

This course does not cover stress management since it is a big subject which deserves to be covered in a separate course. If you have a client who is experiencing stress-related issues consider referring him or her to a specialist coach, psychologist or stress counsellor.

Following are some tips which you may consider for yourself or if you are a therapist you may want to advise your clients as part of the treatment routine. Make leaflets, create a newsletter and send it to your client list occasionally.

To help yourself or your client identify the causes of stress and ways of dealing with it you might want to ask the following questions:

1. What makes you happy and content? Can you do more of it to help improve your state of mind and health? How do you see it happening in real life? What can you do every day/week/month?

2. How can you change what you are unhappy about? Write it down. Make 2 lists - small changes which you can make every day, and big changes which you would like to make within a longer time (e.g. 3 months).
What needs to be in place to help you make those changes? How can you get it?

3. Follow through with your changes daily - keep a diary, record what you have done. Reward yourself regularly.

4. Don't fret or and don't stop making those changes if you have lapsed. It's human to mess up. Just pick yourself up from where you've left it, and keep going. By changes I mean even tiny little things - for example, rearranging stuff in your bedroom wardrobe the way you like it, chucking

what you don't need, sorting out draws in your desk, taking a walk to the station instead of a bus, etc.

5. Include vitamin B complex into your diet.

6. Exercise - not necessarily in a gym, but do it consistently. Walking 1 hour a day is a great way to deal with stress.

7. Take regular breaks from work to do activities which you enjoy.

8. Sleep helps to relieve stress. Make sure that you sleep enough. It also helps to regulate metabolism.

9. Identify when you eat for pleasure, as a way of dealing with stress and anxiety, rather than because you are hungry.

10. Keep a diary. What can you do instead which will satisfy you, instead of reaching for food?

11. Eating a little more often (e.g. 5 times a day) may work better than consuming large meals in one go.

12. Drink water - remember that stress, acute and chronic, create a lot of metabolites and other toxins in the body, and they need to be flushed out.

13. Detoxification is important since stress causes a higher level of toxicity. It can be achieved by eating lots of detoxifying foods (rich in phytonutrients), exercising, detoxifying procedures (far infrared wraps, for example, are possibly the quickest ways to induce profound deep detoxification through stimulation of the body tissues, and sweating).

14. Take care of your social life. Spend time in good company, with people you enjoy being with.
Have regular treatments - Aromatherapy massage and Reflexology are wonderful ways of dealing with stress.

15. Take care of your environment – physical and mental. Deal with toxic relationships - often the best way is out. Are you happy with your physical surroundings? With what you do for a living? If you have low self-esteem, what is causing it? Outdated beliefs? Past events? See someone who can help you develop a strategy to change it.

16. What is nagging you continuously?

17. What is your most common response to stress? Be honest with yourself. Write it down.
18. See a life coach help you make positive changes in your life. It's good to have someone to account to.

19. Where are you heading? Do you have something to aspire to? It is up to you to identify what you want and develop your plan of how to get there, but you may need help with it.

20. If you don't have big goals that's ok too. See how you can make your days more interesting. Consider taking a

hobby.

21. Most of the problems which cause psychological stress are of psychological nature. However, the consequences of it can and often are very physical. So be your own best friend - don't ignore the signs. Deal with what is making you ill.

Stress is often one of the main causes and consequences of magnesium deficiency, and so is obesity. Magnesium deficiency increases the probability of stress-related disorders and reduces the body defence response. This can lead to devastating consequences - physically, psychologically, socially. Topping up magnesium levels daily - by applying magnesium oil all over the body is one of the most effective ways to deal with many stress-related conditions. Combining such applications with far infrared should be used preferably on a weekly basis. to facilitate not only fast magnesium supplementation but also detoxification.

All of these measures are effective at managing weight on a long-term basis. However, remember that a combined approach is needed to address long-term stress-related physical and psychological issues.

Further Reading

1. Why We Gain Weight When We're Stressed—And How Not To. https://www.psychologytoday.com/blog/the-mindful-self-express/201308/why-we-gain-weight-when-we-re-stressed-and-how-not

2. Stress Management. http://www.mayoclinic.org/healthy-living/stress-management/expert-answers/stress/faq-20058497

3. Childhood Obesity & Emotional Eating. http://www.heartmath.org/free-services/articles-of-the-heart/childhood-obesity-and-emotional-eating.html

Module 5 - Importance of Magnesium for Health and Weight Loss. Magnesium Deficiency. Supplementation Methods.

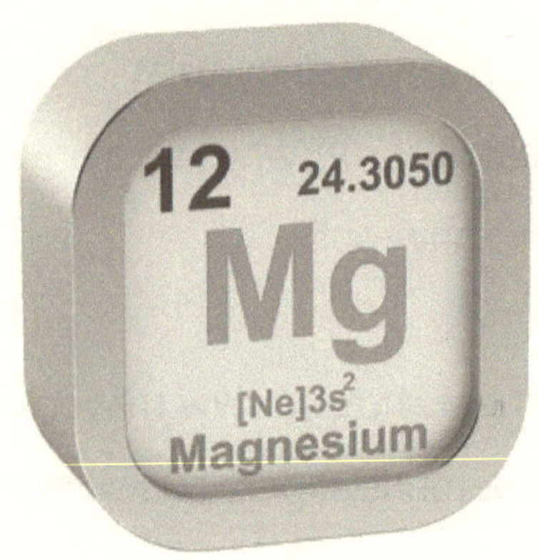

Unit 1 – Importance of Magnesium for Health

Magnesium is rightly called the miracle mineral. There are few elements in nature which attract so much attention.

Magnesium is the fourth most abundant mineral in the body. It participates in over 300 biochemical reactions in the body.

About half of the total body magnesium is found in bones. The other half is found mostly inside cells of body tissues and organs. Only 1% of magnesium is found in the blood where it plays a vital role, so the body works very hard to keep the blood magnesium levels constant.

"...An important participant in enzyme processes which ensure protein biosynthesis and carbohydrate metabolism. It is also very important for the nervous and muscular systems, helps to maintain the healthy tone of the blood vessels. Magnesium is a 'calming' element for the nervous system slowing down the brain activity. It expands the blood vessels and is a natural diuretic. Generally, it is vital for all body systems and processes.

An adult requirement in magnesium is 350-500mg per day. Fresh Green Vegetables, Seafoods, Soybeans, Special

Nutritional Yeasts, Seeds, Apples and Whole Grains are rich sources." Read more about the role of magnesium in the body.

Magnesium has been found to:

- Stimulate protein/fat metabolism
- Support normal muscle and nerve function
- Support a steady heart rhythm
- Normalise blood pressure
- Support the immune system
- Help to keep our bones strong and prevention of osteoporosis
- Take part in ensuring that blood sugar is kept at normal levels protecting the body from diabetes
- Help to prevent heart disease
- Reduce inflammation by lowering the levels of histamine and serotonin (mediators of inflammation)
- Speed up rehabilitation processes in the body
- Increase testosterone levels and sperm production

- Increase metabolic rate
- Slow down ageing
- Reduce cholesterol levels in the blood
- Improve the functioning of the musculoskeletal system
- Reduce blood pressure
- Significantly reduce heart disease and mortality
- Lower the incidence of cancers
- Improve the functioning of the Nervous System
- Reduce the effects of stress
- Increase phagocytosis
- Speed up tissue regeneration
- Improve skin condition
- Speed up body metabolism
- Raise energy levels (magnesium is the essential mineral in the production of energy)
- Promote weight loss.

It has been proved to be a:

- Sedative

- Anti-inflammatory

- Bactericidal / fungicidal

- Circulation booster

- Analgesic

- Immune regulator.

Further Reading

1. Magnesium.

http://www.traceminerals.com/research/magnesium.htm

2. Magnesium.

http://ods.od.nih.gov/factsheets/magnesium.asp

3. Magnesium.

http://umm.edu/health/medical/altmed/supplement/magnesium

Unit 2 – Causes of Magnesium Deficiency

Magnesium deficiency is commonly caused by the following

factors:

- Stress - physical and mental
- Certain medications (e.g. insulin, diuretics, some asthma medications, birth control pills, corticosteroids, blood pressure control medicines, etc)
- Extreme physical training
- Chemical toxins getting into the body from the environment
- Excessive intake of sodium chloride (table salt), sugar, caffeine, alcohol, nicotine, cocaine, fizzy drinks (especially colas)
- Prolonged intense sweating, due to exercise or illness
- Diarrhoea
- Malnutrition. This involves not only insufficient food intake but also the consumption of nutrient-poor foods
- Consuming food products which come from magnesium-deficient soils

- Drinking water which is high in potassium
- Prolonged physical exercise
- Diabetes
- Obesity
- Kidney disease
- Malabsorption - this can be due to compromised levels of enzymes, or unhealthy condition of the gut
- Digestive disorders
- Crohn's disease
- Chemotherapy and radiotherapy
- Liver disease
- Inflammation
- Serious injuries
- Pancreatitis
- Severe burns.

Further Reading

1. Magnesium Deficiency Symptoms & Diagnosis, Mark Sircus.

http://drsircus.com/medicine/magnesium/magnesium-deficiency-symptoms-diagnosis

2. What Causes Magnesium Deficiency?
http://www.magnesiumoil.org.uk/what-causes-magnesium-deficiency/

Unit 3 – Dangers of Magnesium Deficiency for Health

How does magnesium deficiency affect us? Here are the conditions which may develop as a result:

- **Anxiety and panic attacks.** Magnesium helps to keep hormones in balance, and adrenal stress under control.
- **Depression.** Serotonin - the hormone responsible for mood regulation - is dependent on magnesium levels being at an optimal level in the body at all times.

- **Detoxification.** Removal of toxic elements such as lead and aluminium from the body requires the presence of sufficient levels of magnesium.
- **Diabetes.** Magnesium is needed for insulin secretion, to help metabolise sugar. Without magnesium insulin cannot transfer glucose into cells, which leads to the build-up of both glucose and insulin in the blood, leading to tissue damage.
- **Metabolic syndrome.** This condition is partly due to insufficient magnesium levels in the body, which leads to insulin not being activated, glucose not delivered to the body cells, and energy not being produced. This slows down the body metabolism.
- **Obesity.** This is also partly a result of magnesium deficiency, due to malnutrition and slow metabolism. To add to this, there is a permanent cycle of anxiety-triggered overeating, which is caused by and leads to magnesium deficiency. Of course, one cannot just blame a low magnesium level for obesity, but it plays a big role in developing the condition.

- **Constipation.** Magnesium deficiency causes slowing down of bowel movement and constipation, which leads to an increase of toxicity and nutrient deficiency.

- **Muscle cramps.** Magnesium is the ultimate natural relaxant. Without sufficient magnesium in the blood calcium takes over, leading to calcification of tissues and cramps.

- **Musculoskeletal problems.** Aches, pains, muscle tension are all made worse where there is not enough magnesium is present in the body. This happens due to insufficient relaxation of the muscles, which can lead to chronic tension, joint problems, inflammation and other musculoskeletal conditions, such as back problems, osteoarthritis, frozen shoulder, RSA, and more.

- **Osteoporosis.** Blood contains both calcium and magnesium, and a healthy ratio (approximately 2:1 calcium to magnesium) is important to ensure bone health. Contrary to popular belief, just taking calcium and vitamin D, without supplementing magnesium, may worsen the condition, and lead to other problems.

- **Tooth decay.** Insufficient magnesium causes an imbalance of phosphorus and calcium in the saliva, which leads to tooth decay.

- **Blood clots.** Magnesium plays an important role in keeping the blood thin. Magnesium deficiency leads to thickening of the blood, and formation of blood clots, which is a potentially fatal condition.

- **Arterial plaque/ atherosclerosis.** Magnesium is necessary to keep the optimal calcium-magnesium ratio in the blood. When there is not enough magnesium, this ratio gets compromised, leading to the formation of arterial plaque, which consists of excessive blood calcium, proteins and fat. This is also a potentially fatal condition.

- **PMS/PMT** - pre-menstrual syndrome/ tension are often directly linked to magnesium deficiency.

- **Pre-eclampsia, eclampsia, premature contractions.** All of these dangerous conditions are directly caused by magnesium deficiency.

- **Fatigue.** Magnesium is the "energy" mineral. It is the spark needed to convert glucose into energy. Magnesium is also used in the production of a number of enzymes. When there is not enough magnesium in the body, energy does not get produced, leading to fatigue, sometimes chronic.

- **Hypertension (high blood pressure).** Being a natural relaxant, magnesium is needed to keep blood vessels supple and open.

- **Heart disease.** Magnesium deficiency is often associated with heart disease. Doctors have been using magnesium injections for cardiac arrest and arrhythmia for a long time. The heart muscle, like any other muscles in the body, depends on magnesium for relaxation. Where there is not enough magnesium, it goes into spasm, which may lead to a heart attack and other dangerous conditions.

- **Hypoglycaemia** - low blood sugar level. Blood sugar levels depend on sufficient levels of magnesium in the body which is needed for the regulation of insulin activity. Insufficient magnesium can lead not only to a build-up of glucose but to hypoglycaemia as well.

- **Asthma.** Insufficient magnesium in the body increases bronchial spasm, as well as histamine production.
- **Allergy.** There is a direct link between magnesium deficiency and an allergic reaction since magnesium manages histamine production and response within the body.
- **Kidney disease.** Magnesium deficiency can lead to abnormal lipid levels and blood sugar control, which can lead to kidney failure.
- **Headache & migraine.** Low magnesium levels lead to narrowing of blood vessels and muscle spasms, which can lead to restriction of blood flow to the brain. The other factor contributing to headaches and migraines is that serotonin does not get produced in sufficient amounts.
- **Nerve disorders.** Nerve tissue depends on magnesium for its health. Magnesium is needed to

transmit nerve signals between the brain and other organs and tissues since it activates calcium. Insufficient magnesium leads to peripheral nerve problems, as well as dysfunctions of the central nervous system.

These are only some conditions caused by magnesium deficiency. All of them require increased and consistent magnesium supplementation, and oral supplementation is normally not enough.

Unit 4 - Link between Magnesium Deficiency and Obesity

Magnesium plays a crucial part in the production and storage of energy, by activating ATP (adenosine triphosphate) – the molecule which stores energy in the body.

This is what Dr Carolyn Dean, an authority on the subject of magnesium for health, says: *"Magnesium and B-complex vitamins are excellent examples of energy nutrients because they activate enzymes that control digestion, absorption, and the utilisation of proteins, fats, and carbohydrates. Enzymes cannot be produced and nutrients cannot be utilised, which means that energy cannot be manufactured and stored in the body without magnesium."*

Magnesium deficiency is closely associated with obesity and related conditions. Type 2 diabetes is one such condition which is on the rise both in the developed and developing the world. It has been established that type 2 diabetes responds very well to magnesium supplementation. Magnesium is needed for production and utilisation of insulin by the cells.

"Low magnesium, widely recognised as a marker for diabetes, occurs in up to 40% of diabetic patients. Lack of magnesium increases the risk of cardiovascular disease, eye symptoms, and nerve damage in diabetics, whereas supplementation can prevent them. Most importantly for diabetics, magnesium is a necessary cofactor in the production of energy from sugar stores in the muscles and

liver." (The Miracle of Magnesium, Carolyn Dean, M.D., N.D.).

Magnesium deficiency also creates cellular resistance to insulin, since insulin opens the cells to glucose only in the presence of sufficient magnesium, so the cell does not receive glucose, and cannot produce energy. The glucose, in this case, accumulates in the blood causing irrevocable damage to the body organs, blood vessels, nerves and other systems.

Since obesity is often interlinked with diabetes and pre-diabetic conditions, it is very important to ensure sufficient magnesium intake to address obesity and for management and prevention of diabetes. Of course, magnesium alone will not solve the problem of obesity. A lot of factors, such as correct nutrition, exercise, psychological problems need to be addressed. However, if magnesium deficiency is not addressed all these measures may produce only a limited and short-lived result.

As well as eating traditionally magnesium-rich foods, magnesium needs to be supplemented both orally and transdermally in order to produce a visible impact. Spraying or rubbing magnesium chloride solution all over the body on a daily basis, taking magnesium baths or even foot baths can replenish magnesium levels quickly, with powerful results which can be evident even within a number of days.

One of the most powerful ways to administer magnesium is by using a far-infrared sauna and magnesium oil (Magnesium Wrap). It ensures that magnesium is absorbed by the body in the shortest possible time. It also promotes detoxification as a result of profuse sweating speeding up blood circulation and metabolism.

Further Reading

1. Magnesium - the Weight Loss Cure.
http://www.naturalnews.com/036049_magnesium_weight_loss_cure.html

2. Magnesium, Leptin & Obesity, Dr Sircus.
http://drsircus.com/medicine/magnesium/magnesium-
leptin-obesity

3. Magnesium for Weight Loss. http://www.med-
health.net/Magnesium-For-Weight-Loss.html

Unit 5 - Magnesium Supplementation Methods

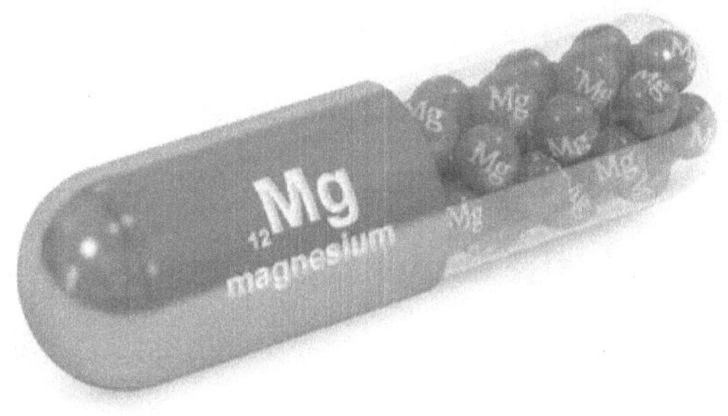

Magnesium supplementation methods

Magnesium can be supplemented in 3 main ways: orally
(tablets, milk of magnesia, capsules, powder, salt),

intravenously (by injection), and transdermally (through the skin).

Some people find it difficult to tolerate oral magnesium, due to problems with their digestive system and resulting inability to absorb magnesium through intestinal walls. With magnesium being a laxative, much of it is excreted without any benefit to the body. Still, it is a method most people use - including me (alongside the transdermal one).

For those who do use oral supplements, please make sure that you use chelated magnesium - not magnesium oxide since it gets into the body in an ionic form, so does not use hydrochloric acid in the stomach to break it down.

Intravenous magnesium supplementation is something which is mainly practised in a hospital environment when magnesium needs to be supplemented quickly. However, it is not a practical method for a home environment, so we won't go into detail about it.

Ways of Dealing with Magnesium Deficiency

- Ensure that you eat plenty of magnesium-rich foods (dark leafy greens, nuts, fish, seafood, beans, lentils, avocados, dried fruit, eggs, bananas, dark chocolate).
- Learn to be flexible in your approach to life situations. Adaptability is very important in effective stress management. Stress is the major contributor to magnesium deficiency.
- Avoid alcohol – it is possibly the biggest "thief" of this vital mineral.
- Avoid tobacco.
- If pregnant or breastfeeding – increase your intake of magnesium.
- Cramps and spasms are an indicator of magnesium deficiency – increase its intake.
- Oral supplementation: use chelated forms of magnesium (magnesium citrate, magnesium orotate, etc.). Magnesium oxide is a poorly absorbed form of magnesium.

The best way to supplement magnesium is by applying it transdermally – rubbing magnesium oil on the skin, taking magnesium baths, foot baths, and of course in the form of transdermal magnesium wraps.

Transdermal Supplementation - Why Choose it?

Supplementing magnesium transdermally is the most effective and practical way to get it into the body. There are simple reasons for its effectiveness:

- The skin is a highly permeable organ, so can absorb magnesium ions from the salt.
- It bypasses the digestive tract.
- It delivers magnesium to the body very quickly.
- Since it delivers magnesium by the process of osmosis, there is no possibility of overdosing on it.
- No special tools or skills are needed for transdermal supplementation.
- There are no side-effects from it.

- Benefits are experienced very quickly.

Magnesium Chloride or Magnesium Sulphate?

I have been asked many times about the differences between magnesium chloride and magnesium sulphate, commonly known as Epsom Salts. There is a great article about it written by Dr Mark Sircus, a well-known and recognised researcher of magnesium and its benefits.

I quote: "According to Daniel Reid, author of The Tao of Detox, magnesium sulfate, commonly known as Epsom salts, is rapidly excreted through the kidneys and therefore difficult to assimilate. This would explain in part why the effects of Epsom salt baths do not last long and why you need more magnesium sulfate in a bath than magnesium chloride to get similar results. Magnesium chloride is easily assimilated and metabolized in the human body. However, Epsom salts are used specifically by parents of children with autism because of the sulfate, which they are usually deficient in, sulfate is also crucial to the body and is wasted in the urine of autistic children.

For cellular detoxification and tissue purification, the most effective form of magnesium is magnesium chloride, which has a strong excretory effect on toxins and stagnant energies stuck in the tissues of the body, drawing them out through the pores of the skin. This is a powerful hydrotherapy that draws toxins from the tissues, replenishes the "vital fluid" of the cells and restores cellular magnesium to optimum levels. Magnesium Chloride is environmentally safe and is used around vegetation and in agriculture. It is not irritating to the skin at lower concentrations and is less toxic than common table salt.

Magnesium Chloride solution was not only harmless for tissues, but it had also a great effect on leucocytic activity and phagocytosis; so, it was perfect for external wounds treatment."

I would add here that transdermally either of these salts can be used to great effect. Magnesium chloride has a lighter structure and penetrates the skin more easily. However, magnesium helps to draw organic toxins from the body due to the sulphur element in it.

Magnesium Products to Use for Transdermal Supplementation

Magnesium oil

Magnesium oil is a highly concentrated salt solution which is not an oil technically but feels like a light oil to touch. Due to its oily consistency, it can be easily spread on the body. The best magnesium oil is the one which is produced from the salt mined from ancient underground deposits. The most well-known source is the Zechstein underground deposit which covers a big area in Europe and Russia. There are 3 main sources of magnesium oil – Holland, Russia and Ukraine. The Russian/ Ukrainian oil is often called "Bishofit".

Magnesium Gel

This is a derivative of magnesium oil, with a gel element in it. It is less concentrated than the oil and is, therefore, milder on the skin. Magnesium gel is suitable for people with sensitive skin prone to irritations.

Magnesium Flake

Magnesium flake is crystallised magnesium chloride. It still contains water - this is why it is called Magnesium Chloride Hexahydrate - but in a much slammer concentration than magnesium oil.

You can make magnesium oil from a flake. Mix 1 part of magnesium flake with 1 part of hot water. If the flake won't mix, warm up the mixture, and add more water. Alternatively, use it in a bath/ foot bath.

Epsom Salt

It is another name for Magnesium Sulphate. Epsom salt can be used in a bath, foot bath, or body wrap.

Ways to Supplement Magnesium Transdermally

- Applying magnesium oil on the body by hand
- Spraying magnesium oil on the body
- Bath - with magnesium chloride or magnesium sulphate
- Footbath
- Compress
- Body wrap.

Further Reading

1. How to Replenish Magnesium Level in the Body & Keep It High. http://www.magnesiumoil.org.uk/how-to-replenish-magnesium-level-in-the-body-quickly-keep-it-high/

2. Magnesium Oil Massage. http://www.magnesiumoil.org.uk/magnesium-oil-massage/

3. Magnesium Oil Compress.

http://www.magnesiumoil.org.uk/magnesium-chloride-compress/

4. The Principle & Practice of Transdermal Magnesium Therapy.

http://www.naturalnews.com/024142_skin_medicine_magnesium.html

Module 6 - Clays - How They Work. Their Role in Detoxification. Types of Clay. Choosing Clay for Detox.

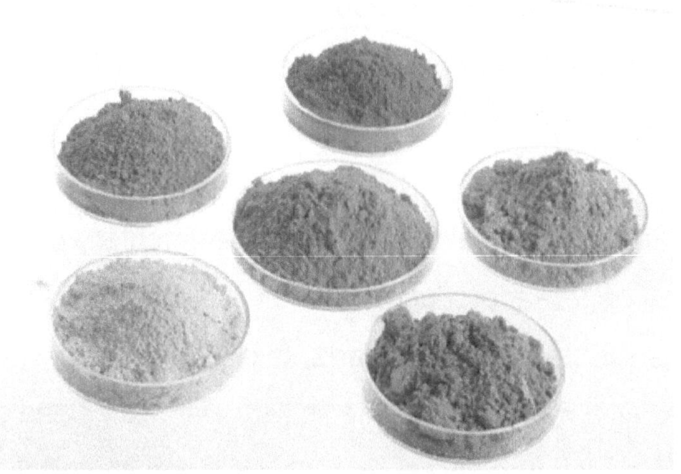

Unit 1 - Clays - How They Work. Their Properties & Role in Detoxification.

Clays are a natural source of minerals. They have been used by all living creatures to cope with various health problems since prehistoric times. Animals eat it and roll in mud –to remain healthy and parasite-free.

Health spas use clays in baths, body wraps, body scrubs, masks, compresses, poultices, for a restoration of health and vitality, as well as in beauty treatments - for skin rejuvenation, detox, weight loss, and as natural ingredients to make own products.

Clays are soft mineral substances of sedimentary or residual origin - a product of weathered volcanic ash. Various silicate minerals (quartz, micas, feldspars) which formed as a result of volcanic activity were subjected to environmental influences, both physical and chemical, and changed into clays over a long time.

Clays consist of minute particles which can absorb large amounts of water. As a result, clays can be hydrated, and some clays expand on hydration. We will talk about expanding clays in more detail later.

Clays are hydrous aluminium phyllosilicates formed from other silicate minerals such as feldspars and micas in the process of physical and chemical alteration and weathering over billions of years.

Most clays are products of chemical or physical weathering which includes hydrolysis, leaching, oxidation, dehydration, temperature factors (heat, frost), animal activity, etc.

The chemical weathering occurs under the influence of weak carbonic acid and other diluted solvents which migrate through the weathering rock. They and are main constituents of sedimentary rocks – mudrocks, shales and claystones.

They can also be of residual deposition and are also main constituents of soils. Some clays are formed as a result of hydrothermal activity. Clay deposits are often associated with a large lake and marine environments.

There are various clay groups, depending on their origin,

chemical composition and properties. The main ones are kaolinite, smectite, illite and chlorite.

1. **Kaolinite** is a white mineral formed as a result of the alteration of aluminium silicates, especially feldspars. Illite has the same constituents as kaolinite, as well as potassium. It is the main mineral of clay sediments, mudstones, and shales.

2. **Illite** is a weathering product of feldspars and other silicates.

3. **Smectite** group has the same constituents as kaolinite plus sodium and magnesium. It is derived from alteration and weathering of rocks. Montmorillonite and bentonite clays are the main representatives of this group of clays.

4. **Chlorite** is not a group which is of interest to us in terms of health and beauty applications, so we will leave it to geologists.

There are various properties clays possess which make them play a very important part in health maintenance:

1. Clays consist of **minute particles below 2 µm in size**, which means that their surface area is enormous and is made many times larger in certain (smectite) clays on hydration. The expanded surface area means that the absorption and ion exchange area in clays is very large – a very important property for detoxification and mineral exchange.

2. Clays have a well-researched ability to **exchange their ions** for those of the surrounding medium. This property is used in various industries, as well as in clay applications for health purposes playing a crucial part in detoxification, re-mineralisation, etc.

3. **Expansion** – some clays can expand on hydration. This increases the surface area manifold, which makes them attract even more toxic substances through ion exchange. Clays which expand on hydration are mainly smectites. One

of the most well-known expanding minerals is montmorillonite, and some clays have a high content of it (e.g. Green Montmorillonite).

4. Clays can **adsorb and absorb** the mineral and organic substances. This property is explained by the electric charge created between the clay layers and on the edges of the particles. This makes them adsorb/absorb heavy and radioactive metals, free radicals, other unwanted products of metabolic activity.

5. **Selectivity** – clays are selective as to what size ions they adsorb. Large multivalent ions (e.g. Cs) are preferred to smaller uni- or bi-valent ions (e.g. Li). This property is used in neutralising heavy and radioactive ions in the environment and the body.

6. Clays act as **catalysts** in organic reactions – the property used in reducing environmental pollution and body toxicity.

7. The **antibacterial** property of clays - clay particles are so minute that they can envelop bacteria depriving them of nutrition and oxygen, thus neutralising them (this is one of the theories for clay's ability to neutralise germs). People and animals have been using clays to rid themselves of infectious diseases for thousands of years. This property makes clays one of the best natural antibacterial agents known to man.

"In experiments, the clay killed up to 99 per cent of superbug colonies within 24 hours. Control samples of MRSA (methicillin-resistant Staphylococcus aureus) grew 45-fold in the same period. The clay has a similar effect on other deadly bacteria tested, including salmonella, E. coli, and a flesh-eating disease called Buruli, a relative of leprosy which disfigures children across central and western Africa.

How Do Clays Work?

Water activates clays by creating cations and anions (positive and negative ions), which in turn interact with various surrounding particles, including toxins, neutralising them through a process called cation (or ion) exchange.

Bentonite and montmorillonite clays are best for this purpose. Another way clays neutralise toxins is through absorption and adsorption – illite and kaolin clays have a higher ability to absorb and adsorb toxins and impurities than other clays.

Clays are a natural source of all the minerals which are also found in a living organism. They have been used by all living creatures to cope with various health problems since prehistoric times. Animals eat and roll in them instinctively when they are sick, or even when healthy – to remain healthy.

Geophagy - the practice of eating clay (or 'dirt' as some call it simply) - is experiencing an unprecedented revival these days, thanks to its amazing benefits.

During the First and Second World wars, many soldiers' lives have been saved by using clays internally and externally. Health spas use clays in baths, body wraps, body scrubs, masks, compresses, poultices, for a restoration of health and vitality, as well as in beauty treatments - for skin rejuvenation, detox, weight loss, and as natural ingredients to make own products.

Further Reading

1. Bentonite Clay Provides a Safe and Effective Detox. http://www.naturalnews.com/025854_clay_body_detox.html
2. How to Do a Clay Pack. https://gerson.org/gerpress/how-to-do-a-clay-pack/?gclid=COrbl92JssQCFcHMtAod6SEAdg
3. Bentonite: Public Research Project. http://www.eytonsearth.org/bentonite.html

Unit 2 – Types of Clay

Clays differ in structure and composition. Just like there are no two identical fingerprints, it is impossible to find two identical clays - they come from different sources, and clay from each source has its mineralogical composition.

Also, clays are rarely found as pure minerals. Most deposits contain several minerals, with one group or type dominating the others. A smectite clay may have a certain percentage of kaolinite, illite, feldspars, etc, with montmorillonite being the dominant one.

We will look here at three main clay groups which have practical applications in medicine, health and beauty – kaolinite (kaolin-serpentine group), montmorillonite (smectite group) and illite (mica group). Each group includes clays of differing chemical composition from different sources.

For example, montmorillonite clays include bentonite clays, Fuller's Earth, and varieties from different sources, with common features and certain differences typical of the deposit they come from. The same can be said about kaolinite and illite clays. There are, for example, different types of illite clays – red, yellow, green, white – their chemical composition determining the colour and properties of the same clay group.

The Kaolinite Group

Kaolinite is a layered alumosilicate mineral with the 1:1 structure - one tetrahedral silica sheet linked to 1 octahedral alumina sheet via oxygen atoms. Its chemical formula is $Al_2Si_2O_5(OH)_4$. The most common clay which belongs to this group is kaolin or china clay.

Kaolin is named after a hill in China – Kao-Ling – where it was first mined. It is now mined in Brazil, France, UK, Germany, China, Australia, USA and other countries.

It is soft, chalky, white, pink, yellow, orange (depending on its chemical composition), of sedimentary origin, formed as a result of weathering of alumosilicate minerals such as feldspar and hydrothermal decomposition of granite rocks. Most deposits contain only a certain proportion of kaolinite, with the remainder consisting of feldspar, mica, muscovite, quartz.

Kaolin has a low hydration capacity – it does not swell in water, due to a stronger attraction between the layers since its interlayer charge is balanced, which does not allow the layers to separate. Its cation exchange capacity is also low – normally 1-15 meq/100g (but can be higher depending on its origin and mineral composition), due to a much lower quantity of active interlayer cations than in smectites. It is highly absorbent.

Kaolin applications in health are based around its powerful ability to adsorb harmful inorganic and organic substances – heavy metals, paraquat (commercially used herbicide – extremely poisonous to humans and animals if swallowed), oil, proteins, and also bacteria, viruses (Steel & Anderson, 1972, Lipson & Stotzky, 1983).

Unlike smectite clays, it attracts particles only to its surface (adsorption), and not between the layers, so the particles can be easily removed from kaolin's surface. Due to its adsorbent, coating and bulk-forming properties, kaolin is used in anti-diarrhoea medications (Kaopectate) and stomach-soothing remedies.

The cosmetic industry is its other big user – kaolin is used to manufacture powders, creams and lotions, soaps, mascara, toothpaste, etc. It also makes gentle, soothing, cleansing, adsorbing masks.

The Smectite Group

The smectite clays were formed as a result of sedimentation of volcanic ash in the soil, rocks, seabeds and water beds. They are the most abundant clays in the soil. They are 2:1 mineral type. The most well-known clays in the smectite group are the Fuller's Earth, Calcium Bentonite (the closest relative of Fuller's Earth, with the only difference that the main exchangeable ion in it is calcium as opposed to magnesium in Fuller's Earth), and Sodium Bentonite. Montmorillonite is the main component in the bentonite clays.

The smectite clays have a very high swelling and ionic exchange capacity and therefore a wide range of applications – industrial, cosmetic, medical and medicinal, in the food industry, agriculture, etc. The high cation exchange capacity is explained by the substitution in the structural lattice of the silicon ions with cations creating a strong negative surface charge which is balanced by interlayer cations $Na+$, $Ca2+$, $K+$, $Mg2+$. These cations are exchangeable, due to their loose binding and therefore give smectites a high ionic exchange capacity.

The most well-known clays of the smectite group are Calcium Bentonite, Sodium Bentonite, Fuller's Earth, French Green Montmorillonite, and variations of the bentonite clays from quarries all over the world. Many of these clays are used for medicinal purposes.

1. **Calcium Bentonite** is a non-swelling clay which has double water layer particles with Ca2+ as the main exchangeable ion.

2. **Sodium Bentonite** is a swelling clay which has single water layer particles containing Na+ (sodium) as the exchangeable ion. It swells up to 15 times when hydrated, and this property makes it very useful in the oil drilling industry.

Sodium bentonite can be used to great effect in detoxification, healing of ulcers, addressing excessive body acidity and associated conditions.

Sodium or calcium in the bentonite clays is exchanged for magnesium or iron. All the bentonite clays and Fuller's Earth have a very high cationic exchange and sorption capacity and are therefore valuable industrial clays. These properties also make them highly prised clays in the cosmetics, beauty industries, food and wine manufacture, and increasingly as medicinal clays.

3. **Fuller's Earth** is a bleaching clay similar in structure and properties to Calcium Bentonite, with magnesium, sodium and calcium as exchangeable ions. Fuller's Earth.

Montmorillonite is the principal clay mineral in Fuller's Earth. It may also contain kaolinite, attapulgite and other minerals which explains its variable chemical composition and properties.

It has a variety of applications in the health and beauty industry due to its high ion exchange and sorptive properties.

4. **Montmorillonite Clay** - a variety of bentonite. Montmorillonite is a soft mineral with high expanding capacity when hydrated. It was first discovered in Montmorillon region in France. Encyclopaedia Britannica defines montmorillonite the following way: "any of a group of clay minerals and their chemical varieties that swell in water and possess high cation-exchange capacities. The

theoretical formula for montmorillonite (i.e., without structural substitutions) is (OH)4 Si8 Al4 O20•nH2 O".

5. **Canadian Glacial Colloidal Clay** - a very close relative of bentonite clays. We will talk about it in more detail in the next module.

Montmorillonite particles are extremely small. They take up water between their layers which leads to the swelling of the mineral on hydration.

Montmorillonite also has a very high cationic exchange capacity. Its high sorptive and ionic exchange capacity is passed on to the smectite clays containing montmorillonite – bentonite clays and Fuller's earth.

These properties are widely used in numerous industries, beauty and health care. The ability of montmorillonite to exchange minerals within its structure for environmental minerals and toxic organic substances is a very valuable property used in detoxification of the environment and human/animal organism.

The Illite Group

The illite group is named for the state of Illinois. Illite is a non-expanding mineral. The chemical formula: (K,H3O) (Al,Mg,Fe)2(Si,Al)4O10[(OH)2,(H2O). Illite is a layered silicate (phyllosilicate). The best-known species of illite is glauconite, a green mineral clay.

It is typically found in clays of marine origin. Other colours include white and yellow. Unlike the Smectite Group, the Illite Group clays do not expand when hydrated. It is, however, a very sorbent clay, taking water into numerous pores in its crystalline structure.

It occurs as aggregates of small grey to white crystals. Illite is the product of weathering of muscovite and feldspar. Structurally, illite consists of tiny irregular platelets of uncertain morphology. It is common in soils and rocks of sedimentary origin. Illite clays are rich in iron, potassium and many other macro- and micro- minerals. Alongside montmorillonite, illite clays have very potent therapeutic properties and are used to treat a wide variety of problems.

Further Reading

1. Clays - Colours of the Rainbow. http://www.saltsclaysminerals.com/natural/clays/other_clays.html
2. Clay. http://en.wikipedia.org/wiki/Clay
3. Clays & Clay Minerals. http://www.ucl.ac.uk/earth-sciences/impact/geology/london/ucl/materials/clay

Unit 3 - How to Choose the Right Clay for Detox

The best clays for detox would be calcium bentonite, sodium bentonite, Canadian glacial colloidal clay, green montmorillonite, green illite, blue Cambrian clay. In some cases, where the skin is very sensitive, I would suggest using kaolin clay mixed with bentonite, illite, Canadian or blue clay. There are also clays which come from salt lakes, which can be used with great effect. However, for now, we will focus on the clays I have mentioned.

Calcium Bentonite Clay

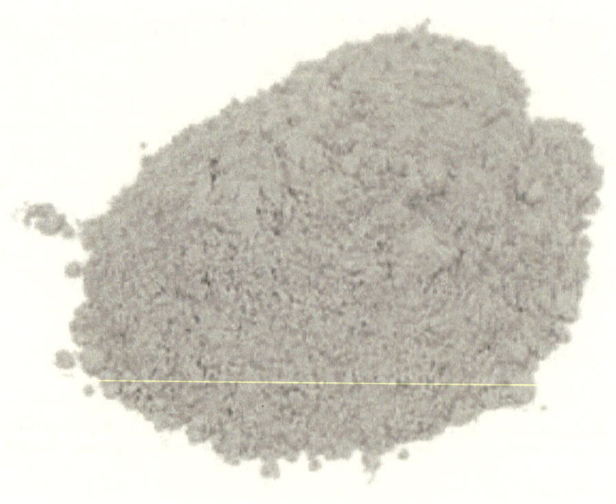

Calcium Bentonite clay is a natural, mineral clay type substance composed mainly of aluminium, silica, iron oxides, lime, magnesium, and water, in extremely variable proportions, and is generally classified as sedimentary clay.

In colour, it may be whitish, buff, brown, green, olive, or blue. In colour, it may be whitish, buff, brown, green, olive, or blue.

Calcium Bentonite Clay has a very long history of medicinal use in all parts of the world, long before it became known as "bentonite", with remarkable results. Its applications in natural medicine stretch from preventative to curative, dealing with such problems as toxicity, infections, and parasites. Research and use of bentonite clays have shown their strong ability to bind free radicals and heavy metals.

For external applications clays are normally used in compresses, poultices, baths, face masks, body wraps, powder applications to weeping ulcers, nappy rash, weeping eczema, fungal infections. They can also be used as tooth powders - calcium bentonite clays are excellent at removing plaque and whitening teeth, due to their bleaching properties (be careful not to over-use it for this purpose, since it can be abrasive and can wear down the enamel). In the cosmetics industry, bentonites are used in soaps, toothpaste, face/body packs, and other clay-based products which are beginning to win the consumer over.

Sodium Bentonite Clay

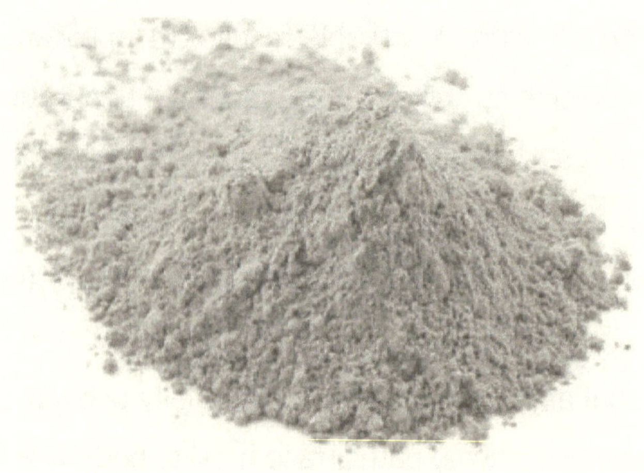

Sodium Bentonite clay is part of the smectite group of clays. It has a 2:1 structure, expands on hydration (up to 15 times) and has a very high cationic exchange capacity, with sodium being the main exchangeable ion.

It is a great clay for treating ulcers, infections and many ailments connected with high acidity since has powerful alkalising properties. The pH of this clay is very high - normally 9-10 – the highest found in any other clay, and for this reason, sodium bentonite clay can be used with great effect for raising body pH as well as detoxification.

Sodium bentonite expands when hydrated, absorbing several times its dry mass in water. This property makes the clay particles expand and increase their negatively charged "active" area many times over. The clay particles become polarised by acquiring a negative charge as a result of hydration. This negative charge, in turn, attracts positively-charged ions called "cations" from the environment. This ability of clays is called cation exchange capacity and is an important factor in detoxification processes since a large majority of toxic substances in our bodies are positively charged. Bentonite clays have the highest CEC among all clays at 70-100.

Because of its high sorptive properties, sodium bentonite clay also works as a magnetic micro-sponge, mopping up what our bodies do not need giving it essential minerals in the process. So, this clay works on the body in 3 ways – by exchanging essential to us ions of sodium for heavy metals, absorbing toxic waste, and neutralising body acids, thus raising pH in a very natural way.

Canadian Glacial Colloidal Clay

Canadian Glacial Colloidal clay is found in the coastal region of British Columbia, this rare deposit of clay contains more than 40 minerals, micro-nutrients and trace elements.

The clay is composed of particles as fine as a mist (the majority are less than 0.15 microns in size), making it one of the finest glacial marine clays ever discovered in the world. It improves blood circulation, detoxifies, exfoliates dead skin cells, tightens up wrinkles, leaving the skin feeling soft, smooth and rejuvenated.

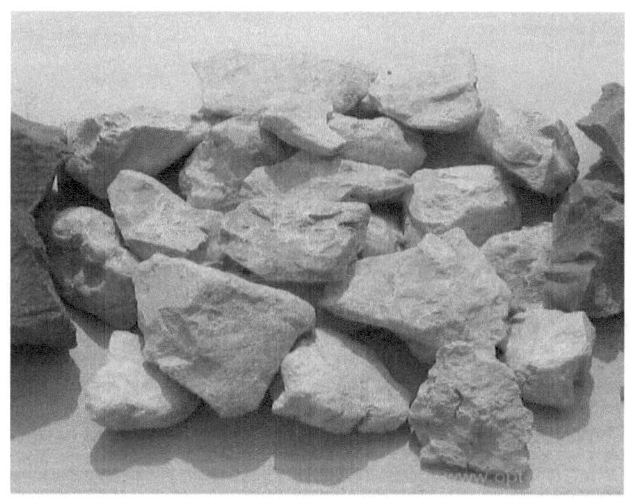

Having a stimulating effect on the cells, it produces local skin warming, accelerates physiological processes and increases cell division in surrounding tissues. It is a perfect balancing and revitalizing agent. Glacial marine clay slows the effect of ageing, rejuvenates tired complexion and renews the elasticity of the skin.

Its microscopically tiny particles have an amazing ability to absorb, and its negative ion charge means that it actively attracts most positively charged particles of organic and inorganic toxins, promoting detoxification both of the skin and body on the deepest level.

For those interested in heavy metal and organic detox, this is one of the best clays ever found in nature for this purpose. Its microscopic particles ensure that the clay works effectively even when a very small amount is used.

To be classified as colloidal, the majority of particles of the material must not exceed .15 microns in size. A cubic inch of these particles would have a total surface area of more than five thousand square inches. This tremendous surface area accounts both for the incredible sorptive action of this clay, and its toxin-attracting ability.

It is profoundly healing. The local grizzly bears and other indigenous animals instinctively use the glacial marine clay and sediments for healing a host of injuries by rolling and laying in it.

In tests conducted over the past twenty years, it has been

found that most clays have a pH factor range from 7 - 14 on the alkaline side of the scale. Glacial marine clay has a pH factor of 6.5 to 7.3, as close to neutral as possible. This is very good for skin and hair applications. In its natural state, it has a moisture content of 35.5%. Unit weight (in its wet natural state) of 109 lb/cu feet, and specific gravity 1.9.

When comparing the percentage of mineral content with other clays, Canadian glacial marine clay is closest to the Delft Marl, which is approximately 50-64% silica and 13-15% aluminium and 4-10% iron. Its microscopically tiny particles have an amazing ability to absorb, and its negative ion charge means that it actively attracts most positively charged particles of organic and inorganic toxins, promoting detoxification both of the skin and body on the deepest level. For those interested in heavy metal and organic detox, this is one of the best clays ever found in nature for this purpose. Its microscopic particles ensure that the clay works effectively even when very small amounts are used.

Green Montmorillonite Clay

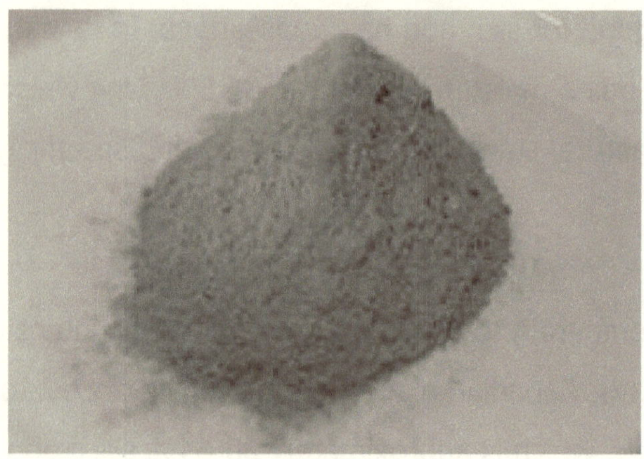

Green montmorillonite clay is one of the most popular and useful clays used in cosmetics and for medicinal purposes. It contains a variety of minerals and salts including calcium, potassium, dolomite, magnesium, silica, manganese, phosphorous, silicon, copper, and selenium. These elements are essential in producing body enzymes which enhance the production of enzymes in all living organisms.

Green Clay - greyish green, the colour is due to the presence of ferrous and magnesium ions. This is the most widely used of the cosmetic and medicinal clays, Green Montmorillonite clay is the best clay for oily skin since it reduces sebum production, works as a wonderful absorbent and an effective exfoliator. It is rich in important minerals and phytonutrients. Good choice for face masks, body wraps, compresses, baths, poultices. It is also excellent for intestinal cleansing programs.

Green Montmorillonite Clay is closely related to Bentonite clay - they belong to the same group of smectite clays. Due to its high ionic exchange capacity, Green Montmorillonite clay is a superb detoxification product. It acts like a sponge, attracting water and toxins not only to its negatively charged surface but also inside its numerous canals, 'trapping' them there via ionic exchange process.

Green Illite Clay

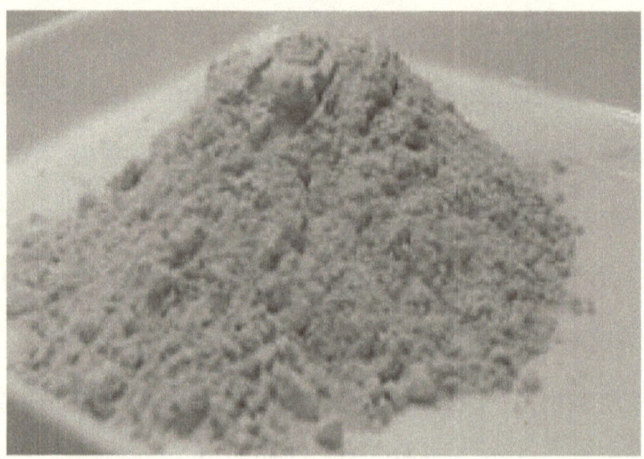

Green Illite clay is the most well-known of the illite group. It is efficient at drawing oils and toxins from the skin and is also often referred to as Green (Illite) Clay.

Unlike Green Montmorillonite, Green Illite is a non-swelling clay. It is sometimes called 'marine clay' due to the quarries being found in the ancient marine beds. This gives Illite a very rich mineral content. It has a better absorption ability than the Montmorillonite - 30% against Montmorillonite's 20%. Its sorptive properties give it a very powerful drying and detoxifying effect. With its very high sorption capacity, illite acts like a magnet for toxins, so it is the greatest detoxifying remedy available in nature.

Recent research indicates that clays can bind mycotoxins. "In experiments, the clay killed up to 99 per cent of superbug colonies within 24 hours. Control samples of MRSA (methicillin-resistant Staphylococcus aureus) grew 45-fold in the same period. The clay has a similar effect on other deadly bacteria tested, including salmonella, E. coli, and a flesh-eating disease called Buruli, a relative of leprosy which disfigures children across central and western Africa.

White Kaolin Clay

White Kaolin Clay - most abundant mineral in the Kaolinite Group - is also known as China Clay or White Cosmetic Clay. It owes its colour to the high concentration of aluminium. It is the most used clay in cosmetics. Due to its natural adsorbent properties, it is an essential ingredient in the manufacturing of cosmetics - soaps, scrubs, poultices, body and face powders, and masks.

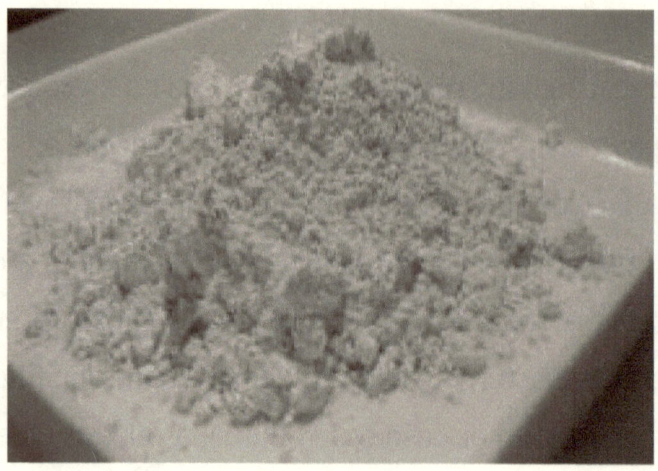

It is the mildest of all the cosmetic clays and is also used as a fixative in the perfume industry. Its action on the skin is very gentle, so it can be used on most sensitive skins. It adsorbs impurities from the skin without removing any natural oils. It helps stimulate circulation in the skin while gently exfoliating and cleansing it. Its adsorption effect is minimal, so it does not draw oils from the skin and can, therefore, be used on dry and sensitive skin types.

Due to its high sorptive property, kaolin has a powerful detoxifying action, attracting to itself ions of heavy metals and other toxic substances.

Further Reading

1. Purchasing /Buying Healing Clay.
http://www.eytonsearth.org/purchase-buy-healing-clay.php
2. Medicinal Clay.
http://en.wikipedia.org/wiki/Medicinal_clay
3. How Clays Work - Science & Applications of Clays & Clay-like Minerals for Health & Beauty. G. St George, Amazon, Kindle.

Module 7 - Far Infrared - How It Works. How FIR Interacts with the Body. Its Role in Weight Loss.

Unit 1 - Far Infrared - How it Works

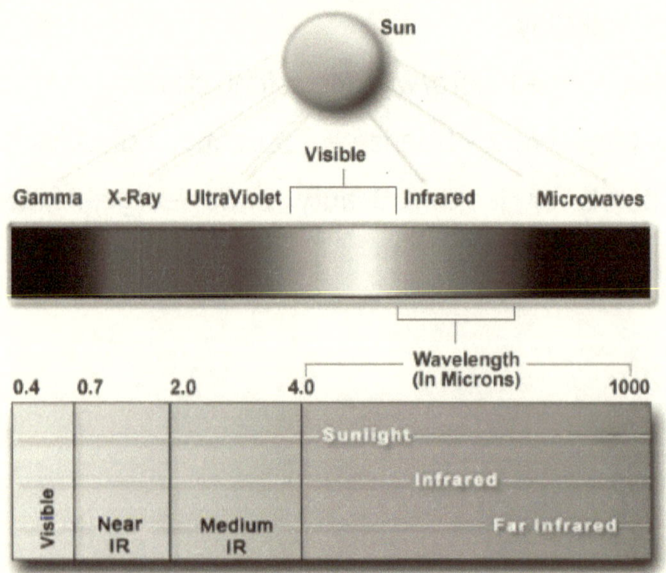

Invisible sunlight

The sunlight spectrum consists of visible and invisible rays. The visible rays are what we can see when we look at a rainbow. They are red, orange, yellow, green, indigo, blue and violet. The invisible rays include ultra-violet, x-rays, gamma, cosmic, microwave, longwave, electrical wave and infrared.

The wavelength of infrared rays is between 0.76 and 1000 microns. Infrared rays are subdivided into Near (0.76-1.5 microns wavelength), Medium (1.5-4 microns) and Far Infrared (4-1000 microns). As we can see, Far Infrared has the longest wavelength. However, only a small spectrum of it is useful to life - the spectrum between 6-14 microns.

Far Infrared rays were first discovered by a scientist Sir William Herschel in 1800 while he was carrying out research; he found that Far Infrared rays were a spectrum of sunlight which existed in between visible light and microwaves. Infrared rays are invisible to the eye but can be felt by the body as heat. It is natural energy produced by the sun – about 80% of it.

Infrared has longer wavelengths than those of visible light - between 700 nanometers (nm) to 1 mm. It was discovered in 1800 by astronomer William Herschel, who discovered a type of invisible radiation in the light spectrum beyond red light, through its effect upon a thermometer. Slightly more than half of the total energy from the Sun was eventually found to arrive on Earth in the form of infrared.

The recent studies have shown that Far Infrared rays emitted at 6-14 microns wavelength played an important part in the formation and development of life on Earth. The balance between absorbed and emitted infrared radiation has a critical effect on Earth's climate. On the surface of Earth, almost all thermal radiation consists of infrared rays of various wavelengths.

Infrared light has many uses - industrial, military, scientific, medical, and others. It is used in night vision devices, thermal imaging devices, astronomy, search operations, weather forecasting. The most important physical property of FI rays is their ability to be absorbed by living organisms and be harmonised with the bio-resonance life force released by the body.

Further Reading

1. The Electromagnetic Spectrum.

http://science.hq.nasa.gov/kids/imagers/ems/infrared.html

2. Far Infrared Saunas for Treatment of Cardiovascular Risk Factors.

http://www.ncbi.nlm.nih.gov/pmc/articles/PMC2718593/

3. Far infrared radiation (FIR): its biological effects and medical applications.

http://www.ncbi.nlm.nih.gov/pmc/articles/PMC3699878/

4. Far Infrared Sauna Therapy.

http://centerforintegratedmed.com/holistic-medicine/detoxification/far-infrared-sauna-therapy/

5. Hyperthermic Detoxification Therapy Using Far Infrared Sauna. Dr John Clyne MD.

http://www.radianthealthsaunas.com/articles-infrared-sauna.html

Unit 2 - How Far Infrared Interacts with the Body. Its Role in Weight Loss.

The body doesn't only absorb far-infrared (FI) heat - it transmits it to the cells, including blood cells, to promote circulation and metabolic processes. Water molecules are affected by FI radiation, with the vibration inside the water molecule being aligned with the vibration of the FI rays.

Since 70% of the human body consists of water, it becomes a superb conductor of this energy, with water molecules in the body getting directly affected by FI rays. We have all tasted the water which we call "fresh". This is what it tastes like when it is affected by Far Infrared radiation. Infrared light is emitted or absorbed by molecules when they change their rotational-vibrational movements.

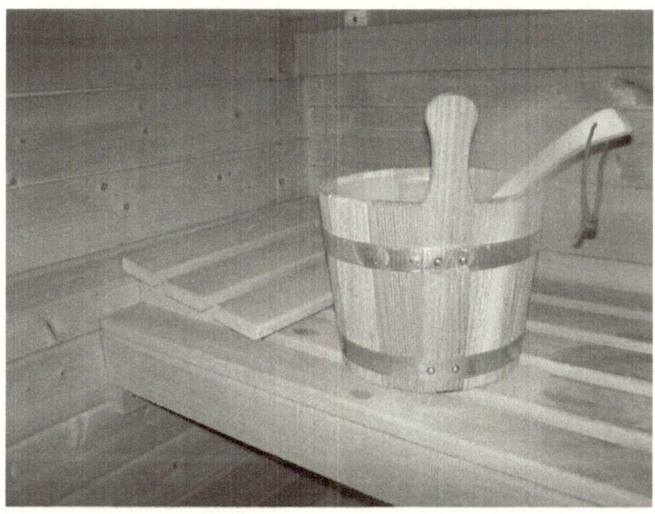

Here is how far-infrared interacts with the body:

- Far infrared gets absorbed by the skin.
- The heat then spreads to the deeper tissues - as deep as 10 inches deep inside the body.
- The affected body cells become energised and activated. This promotes blood flow and metabolic activities inside the body.

Among the whole spectrum of the sun rays, the Far Infrared rays are the safest and benefit us the most. The visible light spectrum, with very short wavelengths, is reflected by the body.

The difference between far Infrared Rays (FIR) and Near Infrared rays (NIR) is that when near-infrared (NIR) waves warm up the surface it gets hot, and the heat is gradually passed on to underlying tissues through conduction. By contrast, far-infrared penetrates deeply from the beginning, so the heat gets deep into the body tissues.

The human body produces far-infrared heat naturally. The intensity of it constantly fluctuates. When it is high, our body functions to its fullest capacity. Low intensity is an indicator that the body is not 100% healthy and that the cells are not producing sufficient energy. This means that we are subject to attacks of illness and tend to age more quickly.

Far Infrared stimulates cellular metabolism which increases

the ability of the body to heal itself more efficiently. It also helps to restore the functioning of the nervous system. When any tissue in the body is exposed to far-infrared rays, the healing processes are activated.

Studies suggest Far Infrared Energy helps to maintain general health and prevent disease. Far infrared rays can penetrate deep into the body, gently expanding capillaries and promoting blood circulation. This, in turn, helps to deliver nutrients and oxygen to the cells and remove toxic substances – organic and inorganic toxins. This helps to restore health and rejuvenate the body tissues inside and out.

Medical professionals in the Far East (Japan, China), Russia, Canada, and other countries are using far infrared systems to rehabilitate and treat various medical problems.

Far infrared heat has been known to sports therapists worldwide for its restorative ability on the muscles and joints. For example, it is used in infrared saunas to heat the occupants.

Far infrared is also gaining popularity as a safe heat therapy method of natural healthcare and physiotherapy. We will talk more about it in the following unit.
The Role of Far Infrared in Weight Loss

Far infrared helps to lose weight for several reasons:

- It penetrates deep tissues, stimulating circulation in deep layers of the skin.
- This increases metabolism, promoting weight loss.
- It also promotes the loss of excess water from body tissues.
- The heat helps to speed up the removal of toxic waste and delivery of nutrients to the body, which promotes weight loss even further.

Unit 3 - Therapeutic Benefits of Far Infrared

Far Infrared energy is very important for life. It plays a vital role in the hatching of an egg, and the development of a foetus of all living creatures. This means the development of organs, the circulatory system, and the formation of new cells. Without far infrared energy body cells simply could not reproduce.

To survive and thrive, a cell needs water, oxygen, nutrients and energy to be delivered to it regularly. It also needs waste materials to be removed from it regularly and efficiently. This allows cells to turn nutrients into energy and building materials for the body - blood cells, hormones, new cells to replace the old ones, etc.

All this is made possible thanks to the circulatory system which acts similar to a pipeline. When there is a blockage in it, nutrients, water and oxygen delivery and waste products removal become impeded. This leads to all sorts of health problems within the body, and in the worst cases - even death.

Since its vibrational characteristics of far infrared are in tune with the those of living cells, it is absorbed by the skin via the process of radiation, going deep into the body tissues, stimulating blood vessels and boosting circulation, which helps to deliver nutrients, oxygen and water and remove products of metabolism, CO2 and toxic waste. The toxin removal function of FIR is very important, and this is why far infrared is used extensively in detoxification procedures.

So, what are the therapeutic benefits of Far Infrared energy?

1. **It promotes the detoxification of the body tissues.** This is achieved through perspiration as a result of warming up of the tissues. To cool itself down, the body releases water in the form of sweat which brings to the surface

products of metabolism and toxic waste. To add to this, an increase in blood circulation leads to an increase in lymph drainage, which plays the main role in detoxification, alongside perspiration.

2. **It speeds up metabolism promoting weight loss.** The warming up of body tissues means that nutrients and oxygen are delivered to the tissues at a faster rate, while products of metabolic activity and CO2 are eliminated faster too. This means that metabolic processes in the cells happen at a faster speed, which in turn speeds up energy consumption. It leads to the body using the energy of fat cells. Since fat cells contain a lot of water and tend to store toxins, the combination of sweating and faster metabolic activity leads to release of both, and this, in turn, makes it easier for the body to use the energy of stored fat cells.

3. **It strengthens the immune system** by stimulating the production of white blood cells. This happens as a result of the tissues being warmed up which speeds up

blood circulation and white cell production. This helps to kill bacteria, viruses and fungi.

4. **FIR heat helps alleviate fatigue**, by increasing circulation and metabolism. This helps to raise vitality & feeling of well-being.

5. **It helps to eliminate lactic acid in the body** which leads to muscle relaxation, alleviation of pain and cramps. This is especially important after prolonged physical activity like sports exercises.

6. **It helps to reduce inflammation, chronic aches and pains.** This happens as a result of increased circulation, removal of toxins, cellular regeneration and healing of affected tissues.

7. **FIR helps to restore healthy pH.** Again, it happens because of an increase in circulation and elimination of acid-producing toxic waste.

8. **It helps to reduce cholesterol levels** as a result of an increase in circulation and metabolic activity.

9. **Far infrared promotes good sleep.** General relaxation involves relaxation of nerve tissues, which leads to better sleep.

10. **It leads to mental relaxation, relief of anxiety and depression.**

11. **It promotes tissue regeneration**, which helps to revitalise the appearance and restore skin elasticity, making it look younger and more radiant.

12. **It helps to keep the respiratory system in good health** and restore it after an illness.

There are many more conditions which Far Infrared can help with. It all comes to its ability to resonate with and work in harmony with the body.

Conditions which benefit from the use of Far Infrared:

- Heavy metal toxicity
- Other types of toxicity
- Lethargy, fatigue
- Muscle tension
- Back pain
- Cramps
- Arthritis
- Aches, pains
- Rheumatism
- High Cholesterol Level
- Diabetes
- Back problems
- Sports injuries
- Respiratory ailments - chest colds, asthma, bronchitis
- Digestive disorders
- Poor circulation
- Poor immunity, frequent infections
- Psychological stress, nervous tension

- Anxiety

- Insomnia.

Thanks to its properties, Far Infrared is used in several therapeutic devices, including saunas, blankets, mats, heaters, lamps, as well as devices for various parts of the body.

Further Reading

1. Health Benefits of Far Infrared.
http://www.clearheatersystem.co.uk/images/health_benefits_of_far_infrared_-_version_21-09-2014_.pdf
2. Far Infrared Sauna, Dr Mark Sircus.
http://drsircus.com/medicine/light-heat/far-infrared-sauna.

Module 8 - The Skin - Its Structure and Functions. The Role of the Skin in Weight Loss.

Unit 1 - The Skin - Its Structure and Functions

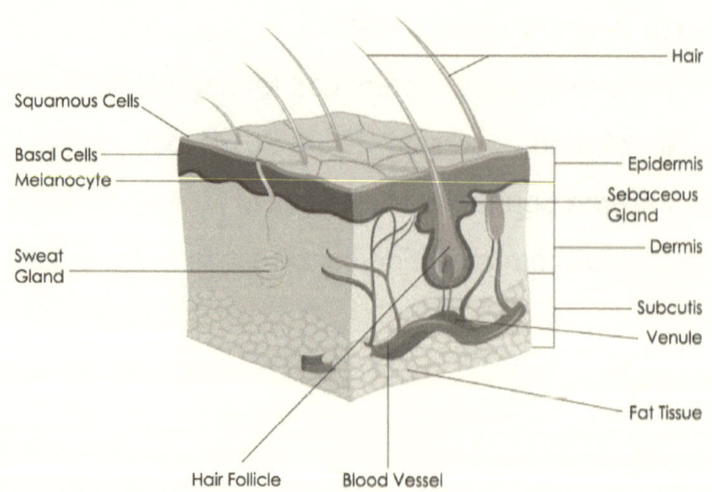

Skin Structure

Skin is a remarkable organ of the body which can perform various vital functions. It can mould to different shapes, stretch and harden, but can also feel a delicate touch, pain, pressure, hot and cold, and is an effective communicator between the outside environment and the brain.

The skin makes up to 12-15% of an adult's body weight. Each square centimetre has 6 million cells, 5,000 sensory points, 100 sweat glands and 15 sebaceous glands. It consists of 3 layers: the epidermis (the outer layer), the dermis ('true skin') and the subcutaneous (fat) layer.

Skin is constantly being regenerated. A skin cell starts its life at the lower layer of the skin (the basal layer of the dermis), which is supplied with blood vessels and nerve ending. The cell migrates upward for about two weeks until it reaches the bottom portion of the epidermis, which is the outermost skin layer.

The epidermis is not supplied with blood vessels but it has nerve endings. For another 2 weeks, the cell undergoes a series of changes in the epidermis, gradually flattening out and moving toward the surface. Then it dies and is shed. Below is a detailed diagram of the skin structure:

Epidermis

The main function of the epidermis is to form a tough barrier against between the body and the outside world, while the dermis is a soft, thick cushion of connective tissue that lies directly below the epidermis and largely determines the way our skin looks. Both layers keep repairing and renewing themselves throughout or life, but the dermis does it more slowly than the epidermis. Under the dermis is a layer of fat cells, which is known as adipose tissue (or subcutaneous fat layer). It provides insulation and protective padding for the body. It also provides an emergency energy supply.

The epidermis consists of 5 layers:

1. **Basal layer (Stratum germinativum)** - this is the bottom layer of the skin. The cells of this layer constantly been reproduced, since they contain a nucleus or seed. As the cells reproduce, the layers get constantly pushed up into the next layer.

2. **Prickle cell layer (Stratum spinosum)** - called this way because the cells have spines which prevent bacteria from entering the cells and moisture being lost. These cells also have a nucleus and therefore reproduce.

3. **Granular layer (Stratum granulosum)** - the prickle cells lose their spines and become flattered. The nucleus dies, and protein is formed called keratin. This protein prevents moisture loss and is found in skin, nails and hair.

4. **Clear layer (Stratum lucidum)** - this layer is for cushioning and protection and is found only on the palms of the hands and soles of the feet.

5. **Horny (cornified) layer (Stratum corneum)** - the cells here are dead and ready to be shed (desquamation). This process speeds up as we age.

Dermis

The dermis is the layer responsible for the skin's structural integrity, elasticity and resilience. Wrinkles develop in the dermis. Therefore, an anti-wrinkle treatment has a chance to succeed only if it can reach the dermis.

Typical collagen and elastin creams, for example, never reach the dermis because collagen and elastin molecules are too large to penetrate the epidermis. Hence, contrary to what some manufacturers of such creams might claim, these creams have little effect on skin wrinkles.

The dermis is the middle layer of the skin located between the epidermis and subcutaneous tissue. It is the thickest of the skin layers and comprises a tight, sturdy mesh of collagen and elastin fibres.

Both collagen and elastin are critically important skin proteins: collagen is responsible for the structural support and elastin for the resilience of the skin.

The key type of cells in the dermis is fibroblasts, which synthesize collagen, elastin and other structural molecules. The proper function of fibroblasts is highly important for overall skin health. The dermis also contains capillaries (tiny blood vessels) and lymph nodes which produce immune cells.

Blood capillaries are responsible for bringing oxygen and nutrients to the skin and removing carbon dioxide and products of cell metabolism (what we call waste matter). Lymph nodes are engaged in protecting the skin from invading microorganisms.

Finally, the dermis contains sebaceous glands, sweat glands, hair follicles and a small number of nerve and muscle cells. Sebaceous glands, based around hair follicles, produce sebum, an oily protective substance that lubricates the skin and hair and provides protection by forming an acid mantle when mixed with sweat.

When sebaceous glands produce too little sebum, as is common in older people, the skin becomes excessively dry and more prone to wrinkling. Too much of sebum, as is common in teenagers, often leads to acne.

The dermis is thicker than the epidermis but has fewer cells. It consists mainly of connective tissue which is made up of fibres of the proteins - collagen and elastin - and a non-fibrous gelatine-like material called ground substance or extracellular matrix.

Subcutaneous tissue

Subcutaneous tissue is the deepest layer of the skin located under the dermis and consisting mainly of fat cells. It acts as a shock absorber and heat insulator, protecting underlying tissues from cold and trauma. The loss of subcutaneous tissue in later years leads to facial sag and makes wrinkles more visible. To counteract it, a cosmetic procedure where fat is taken from elsewhere in the body and injected into facial areas is common these days.

Skin Functions

There are 6 skin functions:

Sensation - the nerve endings in the skin identify touch, heat, cold, pain and light pressure.

Heat regulation - the skin helps to regulate the body temperature by sweating to cool the body down when it overheats and shivering creating 'goosebumps' when it is cold. Shivering closes the pores. The tiny hair that stands on end traps warm air and thus helps keep the body warm.

Absorption - absorption of ultraviolet rays from the sun helps to form vitamin D in the body, which is vital for bone formation. Some creams, essential oils and medicines (e.g.

HRT, anti-smoking patches) can also be absorbed through the skin into the bloodstream.

Protection - the skin protects the body from ultraviolet light - too much of it is harmful to the body - by producing a pigment called melanin. It also protects us from the invasion of bacteria and germs by forming an acid mantle (formed by the skin sebum and sweat). This barrier also prevents moisture loss.

Excretion - Waste products and toxins are eliminated from the body through the sweat glands. It is a very important function which helps to keep the body 'clean' from the inside.

Secretion - sebum and sweat are secreted onto the skin surface. The sebum keeps the skin lubricated and soft, and the sweat combines with the sebum to form an acid mantle which creates the right pH balance for the skin to fight off infection.

I would add one more very important but frequently overlooked function to this list: diagnostic. The skin shows the state of our health. So, when we are ill or otherwise unhealthy, the skin will reflect it immediately.

A toxic, congested, tired, stressed body will often have pale, unhealthy complexion. Deprived of proper nourishment and good oxygen supply due to inefficient circulation and elimination, it will be more prone to various skin problems.

Further Reading

1. Skin Structure & Function.
http://www.merckmanuals.com/home/skin_disorders/biology_of_the_skin/structure_and_function_of_the_skin.html
 2. Skin Structure & Function.
http://courses.washington.edu/bioen327/Labs/Lit_SkinStruct_Bensouillah_Ch01.pdf

Unit 2 - The Role of the Skin in Weight Loss

The skin plays an important role in weight loss since it is the biggest organ in the body which allows both absorption and excretion at the same time which is what transdermal therapy relies on. Absorption allows the movement of substances inside the body and excretion pushes them outside.

Both functions are possible due to the permeability of the skin thanks to its microporous structure. A large number of pores allows the skin to absorb various salts, aroma oils and even larger organic molecules of medicines. This function is very important in terms of transdermal mineral supplementation - for example with magnesium which plays a big role in weight loss.

The same pores also allow the skin to release toxins. Excretion is a process opposite to absorption, with the skin releasing unwanted substances out of the body. Without this ability, the body systems would fail very quickly because they would not be able to do this on their own.

The skin takes upon itself a very important function to rid the body of toxins bypassing other channels, such as the liver and kidneys. This is why in cases of severe skin damage (for example, due to burns), the body systems can fail very quickly - especially the kidneys.

The skin is very large if laid out and stretched, which allows it to work very efficiently. Of course, the skin by itself would be nothing without the network of multiple capillaries take away toxins to the skin surface for elimination. The same network delivers important nutrients from the surface of the skin to the cells inside the body.

Salt ions are easiest for the skin to absorb and excrete, due to their minute size. They come out with sweat and get inside the body when it is sprayed, massaged or submerged in a salty solution.

And here we should mention another remarkable property of the skin - called "osmosis". No matter how salty the water is (e.g. Dead Sea water is over-saturated with salt), the skin will not take more salt than necessary (unlike when salt is taken orally). The skin regulates the intake of salts in a very intelligent way, stopping any salt overload.

This means that saltwater balance is maintained at all times if one relies on supplementing minerals transdermally, as opposed to oral supplementation. No matter how salty the water in the sea, we do not become "overdosed" with salt from swimming in it.

Thanks to these properties of the skin, transdermal therapy is a very safe way to top the body up with the minerals it requires, and releasing toxins, bypassing the kidneys, thus reducing the risk of damage to body organs.

Further Reading

1. 6 Ways to Detox through Your Skin.

http://www.mindbodygreen.com/0-1683/6-Ways-to-Detox-Through-Your-Skin.html

2. Arsenic, Cadmium, Lead, and Mercury in Sweat: A Systematic Review. Margaret E. Sears et al.

http://www.hindawi.com/journals/jeph/2012/184745/

3. Mineral Supplements May Be Used Via the Skin.

http://www.naturalnews.com/010061_minerals_skin_supplements.html

Module 8 - Benefits and Uses of the Far Infrared Mineral Weight Loss Wrap

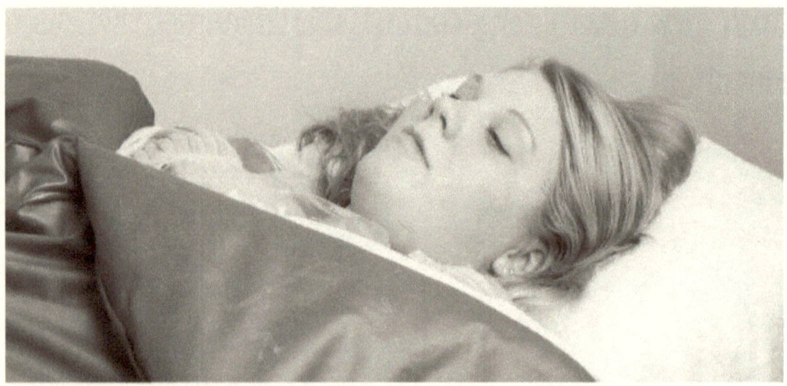

Unit 1 - Benefits and Uses of the Far Infrared Mineral Weight Loss Wrap

Benefits

There are numerous benefits which Far Infrared Weight Loss Wraps can offer. We have already listed health benefits of far infrared heat, magnesium and clays. Used together, they have the potential to produce really powerful results. Here are just some of the benefits of such treatment:

Weight loss

The treatment leads to profuse sweating and speeding up of metabolic activity, as well as higher energy levels. This helps to kick-start weight loss. It should, of course, be used in conjunction with exercise and a healthy diet.

Detoxification

Achieved through activation of the body cells, profound sweating due to far-infrared heat which stimulates the removal of toxins, boosted by the powerful detoxifying properties of the minerals.

Water retention

Lymphatic drainage is activated as a result of stimulation of the blood flow, which helps drain water from where it has been stagnant - mostly the extremities, such as legs and arms.

Skin rejuvenation

The treatment promotes cellular activity and regeneration, which results in skin rejuvenation that can be noticed even after the first treatment. It also softens and hydrates the skin because of sweating.

Stress reduction

The treatment relaxes all the body tissues and systems, including nervous. Magnesium is a powerful natural relaxant, and so is the infrared heat. This leads to profound relaxation of the body and mind.

Sluggish metabolism

The wraps promote cellular activity as a result of the speed-up of circulation. Increased blood flow to the cells helps to deliver nutrients and remove products of metabolic activity much faster.

Relief from aches & pains

Achieved through relaxation of the muscles and nervous tissues.

As we can see, while the focus on these treatments is on detoxification, many other benefits come with it which are certainly worth considering.

Uses

The main focus for the wrap is on weight loss through detox, remineralisation, improved circulation and reduced water retention. However, there are several other issues the wraps can help with, such as:

- Muscle tension
- Muscle cramps
- Osteoporosis
- High blood pressure
- Joint problems
- General aches and pains
- Stress-related conditions
- Fatigue
- Poor immunity
- Insomnia
- Headaches, migraines
- Irritability, anxiety
- Back, shoulder, neck aches/pains
- Sports injuries
- Muscle cramps
- Nervous tension.

Beauty

- Cellulite reduction
- Skin rejuvenation
- As part of a weight loss programme
- Puffiness, water retention
- Body rejuvenation.

Further Reading

Hyperthermic Detoxification Therapy Using Far Infrared Sauna. Dr John Clyne MD.

http://www.radianthealthsaunas.com/articles-infrared-sauna.html

Module 10 - Contraindications and Cautions

Unit 1 - Contraindications and Cautions

The treatment is suitable for most people. However, there are some conditions which would require a medical specialist assessment and approval.

There are conditions which should exclude the treatment possibility altogether, but there are not many of these. These fall into the "contraindications" category.

There are also conditions which should be treated seriously but do not exclude having a treatment. For example, pregnancy doesn't exclude having the treatment, but for the sake of the client and her unborn baby, it's best to be on the safe side and ask her to consult with the obstetrician or GP. The same goes for high and low blood pressure, asthma and other conditions some of which are listed under the cautions heading.

The lists are not exhaustive. If your client has any condition which makes you doubt about their suitability for the treatment, it's best to ask them to check with a medical practitioner first.

Absolute contraindications

These would exclude the possibility of treatment altogether:

- Bacterial or viral infection
- Being under the effect of drugs and alcohol
- Lymphoedema
- Fever
- Ulcers
- Contagious skin disorders
- Scratches, abrasions, wounds
- Shingles/ herpes

- Feeling dizzy and unwell.

Contraindications which may require a GP referral

The following is included in this group:

- Chronic conditions
- Heart disease
- Undiagnosed health conditions
- Epilepsy
- Deep vein thrombosis
- Inflammations
- History of heart problems
- Feeling weak
- Dizziness
- Low blood pressure
- Thyroid problems
- Cancer
- Undiagnosed lumps
- Pregnancy
- Hypertension or hypotension

- Taking prescribed medication
- Rheumatoid arthritis
- Asthma
- Diabetes
- Being on a medication
- Menstruation (it's best to avoid the treatment)
- Anything which you may have doubts about.

Cautions

Treatment can be performed but you should be aware of it and take precautions (e.g. doing a patch test).

- Sensitive skin
- Skin issues
- Acute stages of inflammation (it's best to avoid anything that involves heat).

If a client has any health problems, ask them to consult their GP. If in doubt, do not do it. Make sure that the consent form has been signed by the client before commencing the treatment.

Therapists: what to do if the treatment is unsuitable for your client

It is best to email your client a form before they come for a treatment, to avoid wasting everyone's time. However, even if you do this, you may still discover that the treatment is not suitable for your client. If you find out that this is the case, explain to your client that it is in their best interests to see their medical doctor and ask for their approval for the treatment.

You will also need to let your client know that your judgment is based on their word and that it is in their best interests to tell you everything as it is. Make sure that they sign the consultation form before the treatment.

If you are doing the treatment for yourself you should take the same precautions as you would take if you were doing it for somebody else.

For more information, read this - https://courses.purenaturecures.com/contraindications-cautions.

Module 11 - Far Infrared Mineral Weight Loss Wrap - Consultation (Practitioners)

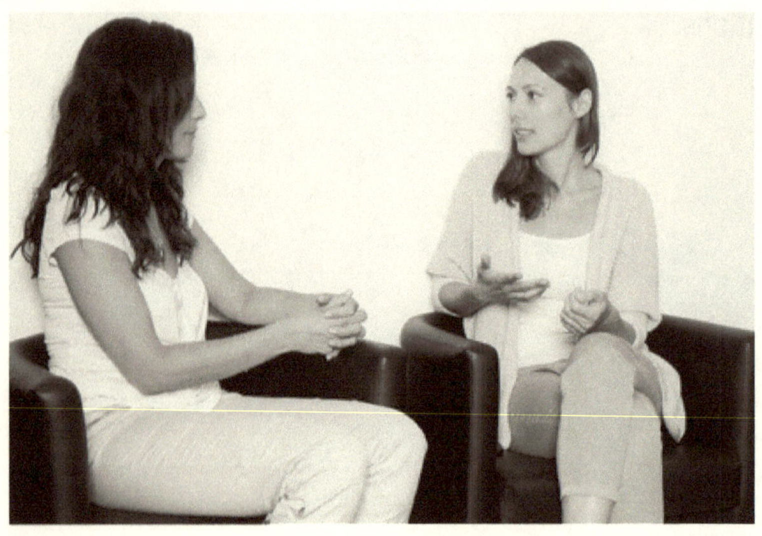

Unit 1 - Consultation

Consultation

- Make sure that the client has no contra-indications by taking a thorough consultation. The consultation sheet needs to include the client's health history, any past or present conditions, chronic or acute, a treatment plan, client's expectations for the treatment (make sure they are realistic), and client's signature of consent to the treatment.

- Check that the client has no fever, are not taking medication or is under the influence of drugs/ alcohol. Make sure that they don't suffer from heart and blood pressure problems (high or low).

- Check their skin condition to make sure that there are no irritations, fresh scars, scratches, inflammations, or open wounds. For a female client – ask again if she is pregnant or having a period.

- Explain what is going to happen and how the client can expect to feel during and after treatment. Tell them that you are going to ask how they are feeling throughout the treatment.

- What is their goal for the treatment?

- Answer questions. Let them know that you are going to stay with them throughout the whole treatment. Ask them to let you know if they start feeling uncomfortable at any time during the treatment.

- Ask the client to sign the consultation form which would stipulate that they have given you all the information regarding their state of health and agree to undergo the treatment. This needs to be done before the start of the treatment.

One of the effects of the treatment is dehydration. Make sure that the client drinks plenty of water before coming to the treatment, and slightly salted water during and after the treatment. It is best to use a bit of sea salt or Himalayan salt to restore the salt/ water balance and prevent dehydration.

Unit 2 – Consultation Form

What the Consultation Form Should Include

- Client's name
- Client's address
- Client's phone number
- Doctor's name and address
- Present health condition
- Past health history
- Your observation of their physical condition and behaviour
- Contra-indications
- Cautions
- What they want to achieve with the treatment(s)
- Agreed treatment plan
- Consent form (disclaimer)
- Date
- Signature.

Make sure that you have all of these things covered, and a get them to sign the statement that they are fit for a treatment - before you commence the treatment. If you decide to do the course a sample consultation form will be included for you to use or to build your form.

Module 12 - Far Infrared Mineral Weight Loss Wrap - Preparation for the Treatment.

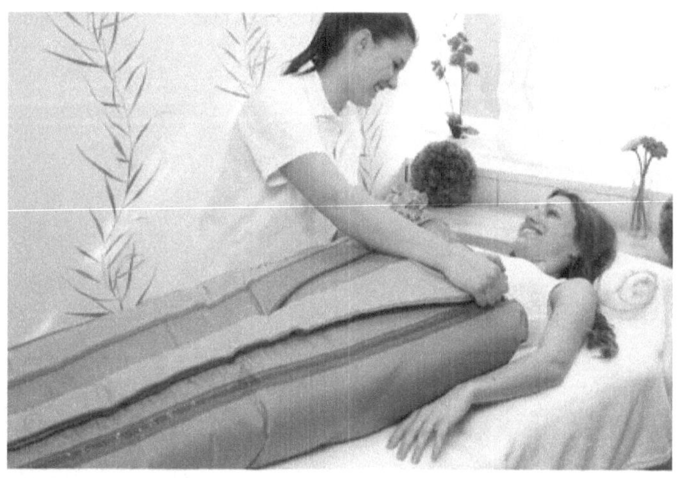

Unit 1 - Far Infrared Mineral Weight Loss Wrap Preparation – Practitioners

Preparation

What You Need for the Treatment:

- Clay/ magnesium preparation
- Massage couch and a couch cover
- Plastic sheet to protect the blanket
- Far infrared thermal blanket
- Large towel
- Drinking water
- Headband
- Disposable panties
- Paper towel roll
- A couch – with the far-infrared blanket laid out and switched on to keep it warm, and the plastic sheet laid out on top of the blanket.
- If you are doing the treatment at home, lay the blanket on the floor or another steady surface.
- Therapists - if shower facilities are not available, as is often the case with a majority of therapy settings, then prepare a large bowl of very warm water just

before the end of the treatment, prepare a bowl of warm water, a sponge and a small towel, to clean up the client after the treatment.

- Set the control device for the FIR blanket on a moderate heat setting and the timer on 30-45 minutes. You may need to reset it when it times out, but 45 minutes will be enough to start with. If you set it 15 minutes before the treatment starts the blanket will be warm for the treatment to be pleasant. Some blankets can overheat in parts, so bear it in mind and if you are treating a client check with them regularly to make sure that they are not too hot.
- Cover the blanket with a thin plastic sheet the size of the client's height. This protects the blanket from getting messy.

How to prepare the clay/ magnesium mix for the treatment

You will need 400-600g of clay powder for 1 treatment (depending on the size of the body being treated). Empty it into a large bowl, add magnesium oil and warm water. Add 100ml of magnesium oil to the mix.

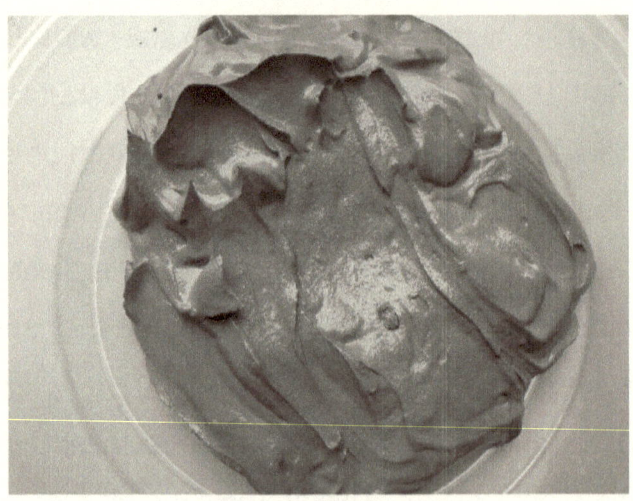

If you are making it from flakes, mix it in the 1:3 ratio (1 part magnesium flakes to 3 parts water) and add 100ml of the mix. Add more or less depending on the client's skin type.

You will need to prepare and apply it straight away to make sure that it doesn't get cold, or if you have it prepared in advance, keep it in a warm place. I suggest preparing it all just after the massage, using hot water which will cool down as you are making the mix.

Unit 2 - Far Infrared Mineral Weight Loss Wrap Preparation - Home Users

Performing the Treatment on Yourself

Is it possible to do the treatment on yourself? The short answer is: yes. How can it be done? The same way as above, except that you will need to do everything yourself, so the process will need to be simplified. For example, massaging yourself would be rather difficult, unless you have someone around to do it for you. So, if you are on your own, proceed straight to doing the wrap.

Materials & equipment

- Far infrared blanket
- Plastic sheet roll (wide enough to wrap yourself in)
- Clay/ Magnesium mix
- Large bowl
- Towel
- Water to drink.

How to prepare the clay/ magnesium mix for the treatment

You will need 400-600g of clay powder for 1 treatment (depending on the size of the body being treated). Empty it into a large bowl, add magnesium oil and warm water. Add 100ml of magnesium oil to the mix. If you are making it from flakes, mix it in the 1:3 ratio (1 part magnesium flakes to 3 parts water) and add 100ml of the mix. Add more or less depending on your skin type.

You will need to prepare and apply it straight away to make sure that it doesn't get cold, or if you have it prepared in advance, keep it in a warm place.

185

Module 13 - Far Infrared Mineral Weight Loss Wrap – Procedure

Unit 1 - Far Infrared Mineral Weight Loss Wrap Procedure – Practitioners

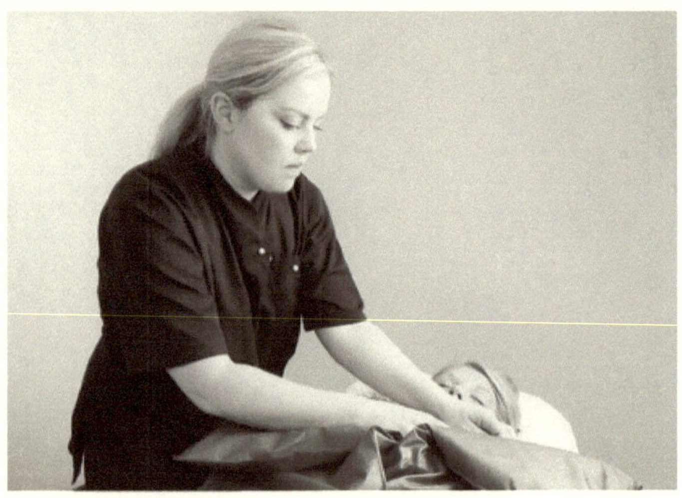

Treatment procedure

- Make sure that everything is on hand to ensure a smooth flow of the treatment. It helps to have a bowl of warm water and a towel in case you need to wash your hands during the treatment.
- Lay the plastic sheet on the far-infrared blanket. This protects the blanket and promotes more sweating.
- A 30-45 minute massage procedure is recommended before product application. It softens the muscles, improves the blood flow which makes the subsequent procedure more effective.
- Use massage oil, aromatherapy oil preparation or magnesium oil.
- After the massage treatment is over it's time to apply the product. Remember that it needs to be warm.
- Start by applying the product on the back, then turn the client over to apply it on the front.
- Having applied the clay/ magnesium preparation over the body while the client is lying on the couch, wrap her up with the plastic sheet she is lying on.

- Cover the client with the top part of the far-infrared blanket. There will be 2 layers in total - the plastic sheet and the blanket.

- If the far-infrared blanket used in the treatment has a zip fastening, ask the client if they are comfortable with the blanket being zipped up. If not, leave the zip undone. The blanket does its good work even when it is unzipped. A blanket with a velcro fastening is the best option - it can be undone very quickly if needed.

- Therapists - always stay with the client throughout the treatment. If you are doing the treatment on yourself, ask somebody to be at home so you can call for help if needed, especially if you have a health condition.

- Make sure that the **temperature is comfortable** for the client. Mid-range temperature provides gentle heat and is pleasant and effective at the same time, since it can be tolerated for a relatively long time without creating discomfort, thus prolonging the interaction of the product with the body. You can lower or increase it depending on your client's wishes.

- **Keep communicating** with the client throughout the treatment to make sure that they are comfortable and not too hot or thirsty. Offer them water regularly. Never leave the room while the client is still in the bag. Make sure that they can open the bag easily and come out of it if they want to.

- The client will normally start feeling warm and sweating 15-20 minutes into the treatment. Normally they will stay in the blanket for 40-45 minutes.

- While in the blanket, many clients want to just go to sleep. If you are qualified in reflexology or are a beauty therapist, you can offer the client a reflexology treatment or a mini-facial while they are wrapped up in the blanket. However, they may just want to lie in the blanket and enjoy the procedure as it is.

Unit 2 - Far Infrared Mineral Weight Loss Wrap Procedure - Home Users

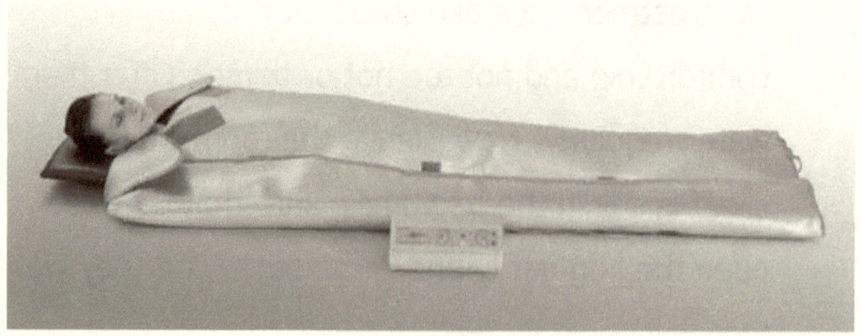

Procedure

- Switch on the blanket to warm it up. It normally takes about 10 minutes to have it warm.
- Lay a plastic sheet the height of your body on it - to wrap yourself in.
- Cover the body with the clay/magnesium mix. For the back part of the body - either ask for help from family members/ friends or spread the clay over the plastic sheet where your back will be.

- Lie down on the sheet, and wrap yourself in it.
- Cover yourself with the top part of the blanket.
- Stay in the blanket for about 40-45 minutes, or less if you are feeling hot and uncomfortable.
- Get out of the blanket.
- Take a shower.

It is good to have someone present while you are having the treatment - to help with fiddly tasks (such as covering your body with magnesium and wrapping yourself in the sheets and the blanket), as well as to keep an eye on you in case you want a drink of water. But if you are in good health, it is not necessary - just an advantage.

It is also good to do this treatment before bedtime so that you can sleep afterwards. Make sure you drink plenty of water afterwards. I suggest adding a small pinch of Himalayan or sea salt to the water, to restore the salt/water balance within the body.

Module 14 - Practitioners - Ending the Treatment, Aftercare, Feedback, Re-book.

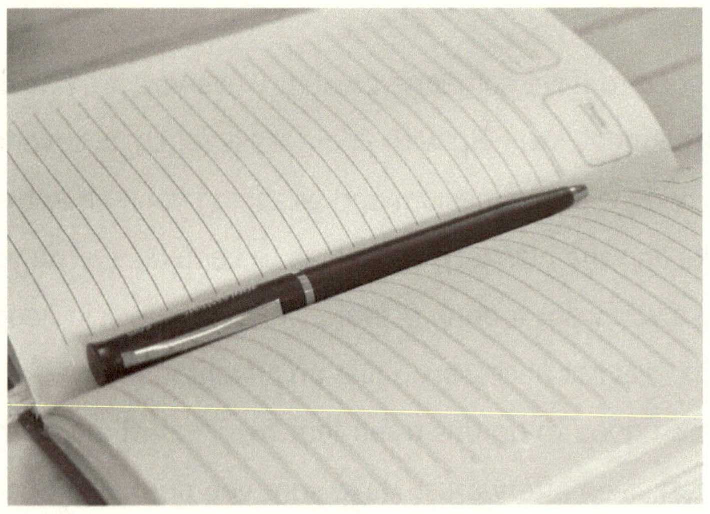

Unit 1 - Ending the Treatment, Aftercare, Feedback, Re-book (Practitioners)

Ending the treatment

- After the treatment is finished, unwrap the client and use a sponge and a bowl of warm water or a small wet towel to remove the clay from the body.
- If you have shower facilities, offer a shower.
- If a shower is not available, use a bowl of water and a sponge plus a small towel to clean and dry the client up.
- Moisturise the client's skin.
- Ask how they are feeling. Make sure they are not drowsy or are otherwise feeling unwell.
- Offer them to rest in the reception for 10-15 minutes to cool down and regain balance before they leave the clinic.
- Offer the client water or herbal tea to rehydrate, and advise them to keep drinking mineral water.
- Clean up the equipment and the blanket. The best thing to do is to wash it up with soap to keep it clean for the next time.

Aftercare, Feedback, Rebook

- **Aftercare advice:** Advise the client to drink lots of water to re-hydrate (slightly salted/ mineral water), no heavy meals on the day, sleep and relaxation are essential. Explain how they may feel after the treatment - light-headed, have a slight headache, feeling tired for a while, depending on their general health condition. Explain that these are normal feelings and that they will pass eventually. Tell them to see the doctor if they start feeling poorly, or are otherwise concerned about their condition.

- **Feedback:** How does the client feel? Did she/he enjoy the treatment? Is there anything that he/she didn't like?

- **Rebook:** Explain that while a one-off treatment is beneficial, the best results can be achieved if they undertake a course of at least 4 treatments, preferably once a week. Offer discounts on block bookings.

Module 15 - The Importance of Correct Nutrition, Lifestyle and Exercise for Long-Term Weight Loss

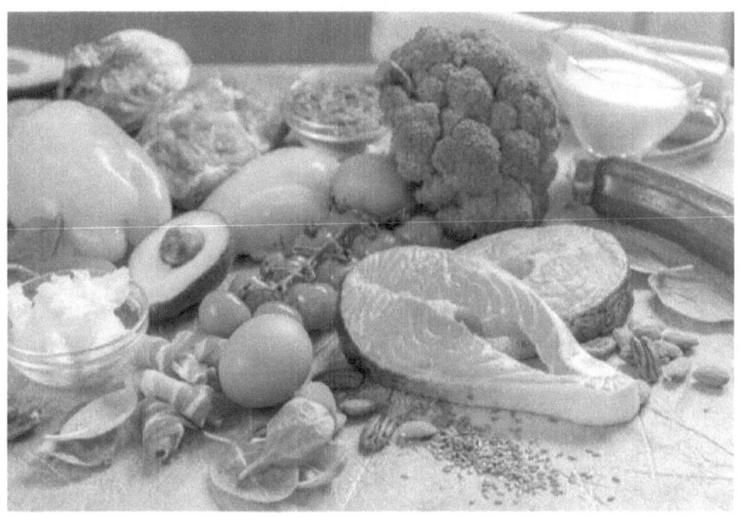

Unit 1 - Tips for Maintaining a Healthy Weight

There are many books and articles written about keeping a healthy weight. Many of them contradict each other and common sense itself. In this unit, I have compiled a list of those common-sense tips which you may want to offer your clients.

Tips for maintaining a healthy weight

- Eat healthily - lots of vegetables, fruit, pulses, herbs, salads, raw food, nuts, sprouted grains.
- Shop for health. Buy the foods which nourish you, not satisfy your cravings.
- Cook at home. When you do, you know what you put in your cooking. You are much more conscious of your choices too.
- Avoid junk food. Sugary stuff, salt-loaded foods, takeaways, biscuits, fried, fatty foods - anything which may look appealing to an eye, but is loaded with the stuff that is going to create havoc once in your body. You need to digest it, and digestion needs a lot of energy. This is one of the downsides

of eating junk - the metabolic rate slows down since the body energy goes on breaking down all those heavy foods.

- Eat less than what makes you feel full while still at the table. The brain doesn't receive the signal that the stomach is full for some time after eating. So, it's good to stop eating with a stomach feeling a bit empty. The feeling of being full will catch up with you shortly.

- Be active (even 1-hour daily walk is good). Aim to do it every day. This boosts circulation, activating all the body processes, which is part of healthy weight maintenance.

- Have a balanced lifestyle. Rest is as important as any other activity, and even more. Do enjoyable activities when you take a break. Don't work non-stop, and don't work long hours.

- Have a balanced approach to life and what it brings. Avoid the aggravation and getting stressed about things. There is no need to fret over what hasn't happened yet, or what has happened, but cannot be changed. Use a constructive approach, or just put it behind you. Get rid of energy-suckers.

- Develop relationships which nourish your friendships, love, family. They all need to be based on mutual respect and benefits to all.

- 10. Sleep enough. It is very important to have a good night's sleep, every night. Sleep helps you recover from the day before, and feel energetic in the morning. This means that you can cope with life mentally and physically.

- Go easy on the alcohol. It does make you put on weight. Alcohol is fermented sugar after all.

- Avoid smoking. Unhealthy lungs mean that your blood doesn't get oxygenated. This means that your cells don't get the oxygen they need, so you feel tired. Fatigue contributes to weight gain.

- Avoid hormone treatments when possible. Hormones disrupt the body systems, and in many ways its metabolic rate.

- Use a natural approach to health as much as possible. Of course, get diagnosed if you feel unwell.

However, too many people start taking medication for symptoms which don't need them. Be discerning, and always seek the second opinion with another doctor, especially if you are facing a lifetime of taking medication.

- Detoxify your body regularly. Use Far Infrared mineral wrap treatments, or the Far Infrared blanket on its own when you can't have a wrap.

- Drink water frequently. 2 litres a day should be the norm. Water is needed to help deliver nutrients to the cells, and take away products of metabolism. Without water, toxins accumulate and get deposited in fatty tissues. This slows down metabolism and makes weight maintenance a much more difficult task.

- Having a healthy body and mind means that you are in balance, and your weight is maintained at its best. Healthy weight maintenance is so much more than just the physical - diet and exercise. It is all of you. It's called the holistic approach. Start introducing it into your daily routines. Change one thing at a time, practice it until it becomes a habit. Then move onto the other. If you get stuck, ask yourself an honest question - why? If you are honest with yourself, you will find the answer.

Further Reading

1. What's the best approach to weight loss? Ten 2014 studies to note. http://www.latimes.com/opinion/opinion-la/la-ol-weight-loss-studies-20141212-story.html#page=1
2. Long-term weight-loss maintenance. http://ajcn.nutrition.org/content/82/1/222S.long

Unit 2 - Weight Loss - What Works, What Doesn't, and What Works, but Is Best to Avoid

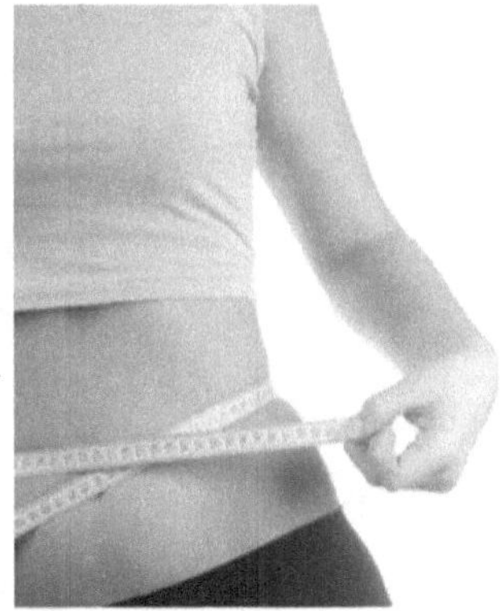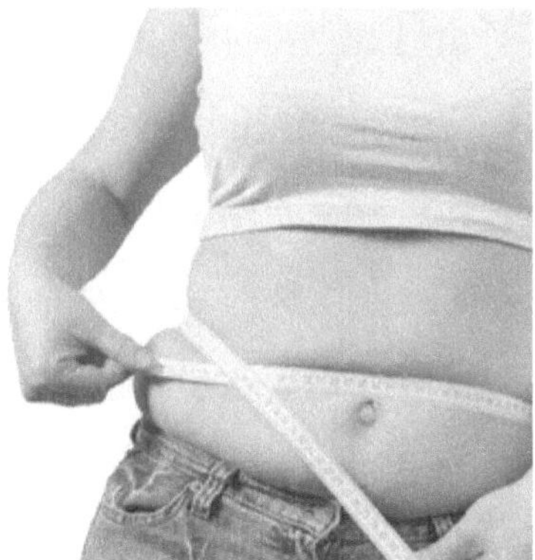

With obesity becoming a worldwide problem and the number of obese people rising fast, weight loss industry is booming. Countless diets are popping up here and there, each claiming to be a new miracle. It's not surprising that there is a lot of confusion as to what works and what doesn't.

Listed are just some guidelines which have proven to work with time.

What works

- Spend more calories than you consume. This is the simplest formula for weight loss, and all the diets and nutrition plans are based on it.

- Sleep enough. Insufficient sleep slows down the metabolic rate.
- Nutritious breakfast is the best way to kick-start your day and metabolism. So, don't skip it.
- Exercise regularly. Walking, cycling, swimming - whatever you enjoy most. Just make sure you do it regularly.
- If you have a sedentary job, get up and have an active break every 2 hours, for 10-15 minutes.
- Cut down your portion size by using a smaller plate.
- Eat more low-calorie food such as vegetables and salads, and less high-calorie food - rich in carbohydrates (especially refined) and fats (especially animal and trans-fats).
- Drink water before a meal. It fills up the stomach, so you tend to eat less during a meal.
- 2-3 healthy small snacks between meals can be a good idea. This will reduce appetite and lead to eating less during a meal.

- Planning your meals is a good idea too since you know what you will be eating throughout the day, which helps with weight management. Plan your meals for a week ahead.
- Shop for health - buy what you are going to be thankful to yourself for, according to your weekly eating plan.
- Avoid buying foods which contain artificial sweeteners and additives. The more ingredients on the package, the more reasons to avoid the product.
- Avoid drinking water bottled in plastic bottles. Plastics have been shown to leach chemicals into the water and disrupt the endocrine system.
- Buy less, but aim for good quality organic food.
- Avoid hormone therapy where at all possible. This means hormone-based contraceptives, as well as medicine-based HRT. Anti-inflammatory drugs - corticosteroids - fall into the same category.
- Avoid sugar and sugary food. People can develop an addiction to sugar. The younger we start, the more difficult it can be to beat it. Make sure that your kids

stay away from sugar, and eat healthy foods from the time they start eating. If you are a breastfeeding mum, stay away from sugar yourself to ensure that you are on a healthy diet.

What doesn't work (at least long-term)

- **Yo-yo dieting.** That's one of the worst things to do to yourself. It does help to lose weight, but then the weight goes up as you stop, since having lost it, you start feeling "safe", and relax in terms of the foods you eat. Have you ever been in this situation? I know I have. And the weight piles up little by little, gradually depriving you of your gains. Then, before you know, you are heavier than before you started.

- **Cutting down on calories, but not increasing physical activity.** The body can adjust quickly to dietary changes. To save itself, it adjusts by slowing down metabolism. So yes, you will lose a bit when you cut down calorie intake while living a physically inactive life. However, the weight loss will slow down as the body gets used to the new regime, due to slowing down of metabolic rate.

- **Reading and following too many conflicting theories on weight loss.** There is no shortage of these in the market. There are so many that it is easy to get lost, especially when one is desperately seeking a solution. However, this just leads to yo-yo dieting and disruption of metabolism.

What works but is best to avoid

- **Gastric bypass surgery** - part of the intestine is grafted on the top of the stomach to create a small pouch to hold food and bypass the stomach. This means that the newly created "stomach" can only hold a tiny amount of food. The surgery is permanent and is available only in extreme cases of obesity on the NHS.
- **Gastric banding** - keyhole surgery is used to tie an inflatable band around the top part of the stomach,

to reduce its capacity and the speed the food passes into the stomach.

- **Gastric balloon insertion** - a balloon is inserted into the stomach using an endoscope, which is then filled with a liquid or air to reduce the space in the stomach and create a feeling of fullness. The balloon is removed after about 6 months.

- All of the above, especially the first 2 methods, **should only be used in extreme cases**. They all have a lot of side-effects - physical and psychological. However, in many cases they save lives. This is why they should only be used where there is an immediate danger to health.

- **Liposuction surgery** - a corrective surgery to address certain areas of the body - like the stomach, hips, etc. The fat is "sucked out" of these areas using medical suction instruments. The effect is temporary, since it is a cosmetic procedure, and if healthy habits are not introduced, the fat piles up again. Besides, being a surgical procedure, it carries a risk of complications, so is best avoided.

- **Drugs which reduce absorption of dietary fat** - like Alli, Xenical, etc. They do work, but the side-effects are pretty abysmal: loose stool, oily spotting, frequent or hard-to-control bowel movements; reports of rare, but serious liver injury.

- **Appetite suppression drugs** - e.g. Sibutramine. While they can reduce appetite, the side effects also include increased blood pressure, dry mouth, constipation, headache, and insomnia.

- **Drugs which reduce the absorption of glucose** - e.g. Metformin. It reduces glucose production by the liver and an increase of absorption of glucose by the liver.

Other weight-loss drugs have also been associated with medical complications, such as fatal pulmonary hypertension and heart valve damage due to Redux and Fen-phen, and haemorrhagic stroke due to phenylpropanolamine. Many of these substances are related to amphetamine.

https://en.wikipedia.org/wiki/Anti-obesity_medication

All of the medications need to be used with **great caution**, and **on prescription only**. Unfortunately, they are often abused by people who do not need them - e.g. teenagers with psychological problems. Even when they are used by people who are in desperate need of weight reduction, these people often have a lot of health issues which may contra-indicate these medications. So be careful what you put into your mouth. And by all means, avoid anything which is promoted as weight loss medication on the internet. A lot of these medicines are unlicensed and can be outright dangerous.

Further reading

1. Weight Loss: Fact and Fiction – What Works and What Doesn't. http://drhyman.com/blog/2013/02/09/weight-loss-fact-and-fiction-what-works-and-what-doesnt/
2. http://www.mindbodygreen.com/0-12901/8-things-every-woman-over-40-needs-to-know-about-losing-weight.html

Module 16 - Case studies and Practical Training

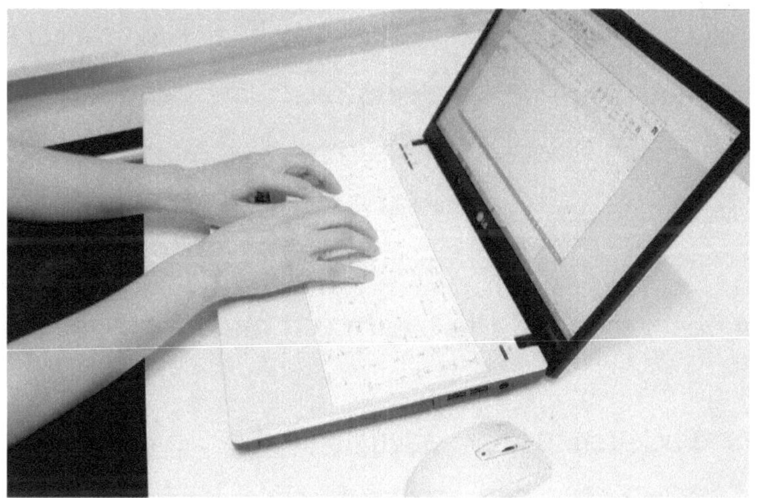

Unit 1 - Case studies and Practical Training

Students who are training to offer therapies to the members of the public will be required to submit case studies on 3 clients (2 treatment for each client minimum) before a certificate of completion will be issued.

The case studies can be performed on family members, friends or other volunteers. The case studies must include a consultation form with a client's real name, address, signature and feedback. The case studies can be submitted by post, in person, or online.

The description of the treatment must include:

- Background information about the client - name, age, gender, occupation, lifestyle.
- Her/his physical condition.
- Their psychological state.
- Their goal for the treatment.
- Any existing contra-indications.
- What treatment plan has been agreed with them (how many treatments, how often, how long, what will be the focus on for the treatments).
- How each treatment went.

- How the client felt before, during and after the treatment.
- Client's feedback.
- Aftercare advice is given.

Each treatment should be recorded separately. You will need to conduct at least 2 treatments per client, 3 clients in total for certification. At the end of the course of treatments, you will need to record a general conclusion as to whether the goals for the course of treatments have been achieved. There should also be a general signed consultation form (one is enough) for the course of treatments.

If you decide to do the online course you will be provided with the sample case study description and consultation form. This is not a certifiable version of the course, but if you would like to access the sample case study please get in touch with us and we will send the details to you.

Units 2-3

These units contain a sample consultation form and an upload area for the case studies. If you decide to do the online course you will have access to both units. The same applies here – you can get access to the consultation form if you would like to see it by getting in touch with us.

Unit 4

Natural Health Practitioners will need to take a short add-on course in addition to the main course as well as the practical training module to get qualified. The Practical Module is optional since it involves face-to-face training and many of our students are unable to do it due to the geographical factors.

We strongly advise UK/Northern Ireland practitioners to do it since it gives better chances of understanding what is involved, an opportunity to ask questions while doing the module and an improved confidence as practitioners.

Our students in other countries need to make enquiries and arrangements locally regarding professional insurance, and of course, for you, the Practical module is an option.

Although for non-therapists the practical module is an option, we suggest that you take it for a better understanding of the procedures, and to get answers to any questions you may have while learning it.

The duration of the training is 4-6 hours. It is normally conducted in the groups of 2-4 people, but we may increase the group sizes in the future. You can either bring your model for the treatment or work on each other. Materials and equipment will be provided for practical training, so you don't need to bring anything for it - just a notebook and a pen.

Further Information

Did you find information in this book useful? Leave feedback to me know what you think! Would you like to learn more? I have published a number of books on the subject of minerals. You can find them on Amazon.

Mineral Healing Books

1. **Earth's Humble Healers:** Learn How to Use Salts, Muds & Clays for Better Health, Youth & Vitality. Plus 80 Health & Beauty Recipes

2. **How Clays Work:** Science & Applications of Clays & Clay-like Minerals in Health & Beauty

3. **Magnesium at Home:** 25 Most Common Health Conditions & How Magnesium Salts Can Help

4. **Mineral Healing Recipe Book:** An overview of how minerals can be used in everyday life to address common health problems, boost health and vitality.

5. **Introduction to Mineral Healing**

Learn interesting facts about healing properties of salts,

muds, clays, zeolite and diatomaceous earth. It is a good book to start learning about minerals.

6. **<u>First Aid Guide to Minerals</u>**

Find out how salts, muds and clays can help when medicines are unavailable.

Courses

1. **Far Infrared Mineral Weight Loss Wrap Course** for Clinic & Home Use: Learn how to use clays, salts and far infrared for sustainable weight loss and better health
https://www.amazon.com/dp/B07N99H1XV

2. **Far Infrared Magnesium Wrap Course for Clinic & Home Use**: Learn how to use magnesium salts and far infrared for better health and vitality
https://www.amazon.com/dp/B07JZDWQX1

3. **Transdermal Magnesium Therapy Course for Clinic & Home Use**
https://www.amazon.com/dp/B07GXXGWT7

4. Far Infrared Clay Detox Wrap Course for Clinic & Home Use: Learn how to use clays and far infrared for transdermal detox and healing

https://www.amazon.com/dp/B07JCL55TZ

5. Forever Young: Far Infrared Remineralising & Rejuvenating Seaweed Wrap Course: Learn how to use the power of the sun, the earth & the ocean to stay young, vibrant and healthy

https://www.amazon.com/dp/B097CWDCG4

If you prefer to read books in the **PDF format**, you can buy them here:

https://purenaturecures.com/book-shop

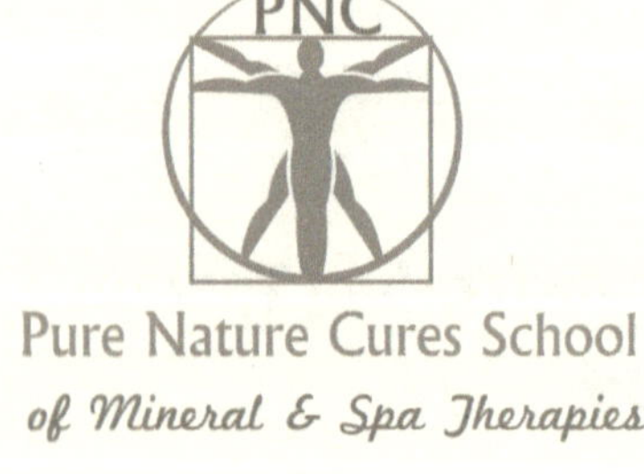

Pure Nature Cures School
of Mineral & Spa Therapies